My
Happy
Mind

For Oscar and Bella, who've brought me unimaginable joy, love and laughter and who inspire me every single day.

LAURA EARNSHAW

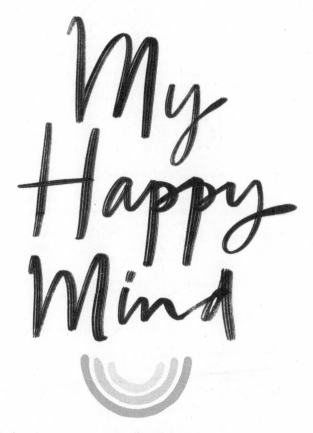

My
Happy
Mind

Help your child build lifelong confidence and resilience

Vermilion
LONDON

3

Published in 2020 by Vermilion, an imprint of Ebury Publishing,
20 Vauxhall Bridge Road,
London SW1V 2SA

Vermilion is part of the Penguin Random House group of companies
whose addresses can be found at global.penguinrandomhouse.com

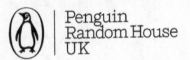

Penguin
Random House
UK

First published in the United Kingdom by Vermilion in 2020

www.penguin.co.uk

A CIP catalogue record for this book is available from the British Library

ISBN 9781785043376

Printed and bound in Great Britain by Clays Ltd, Elcograf S.p.A.

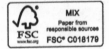

MIX
Paper from
responsible sources
FSC® C018179

Penguin Random House is committed to a
sustainable future for our business, our readers
and our planet. This book is made from Forest
Stewardship Council® certified paper.

The information in this book has been compiled by way of general guidance in
relation to the specific subjects addressed. It is not a substitute and not to be relied
on for medical, healthcare, pharmaceutical or other professional advice on specific
circumstances and in specific locations. Please consult your GP before changing,
stopping or starting any medical treatment. So far as the author is aware the
information given is correct and up to date as at August 2020. All names in cases
studies have been changed. Practice, laws and regulations all change, and the
reader should obtain up to date professional advice on any such issues. The author
and publishers disclaim, as far as the law allows, any liability arising directly or
indirectly from the use, or misuse, of the information contained in this book.

Contents

Preface

'He just needs to develop a stiff upper lip. If he could just man up a little bit, he'd be fine.'

The *Cambridge Dictionary* defines a stiff upper lip as: 'Someone who has a stiff upper lip does not show their feelings when they are upset.' And to 'man up a little bit' means that the person 'should deal with something more bravely'.

This was the response from my child's school when I asked the question, 'What can we do to better support my four-year-old, who is clearly struggling emotionally?'

I'd gone in to see the school because I knew my son needed some additional support. Every morning at drop-off he'd cry and hang on to my leg for dear life, begging me not to send him in. I was that mum who, when it was time for pick up, the teacher would pull me to one side to tell me he'd had another unsettled day. He'd have those heartbreaking red bags under his eyes because he'd been crying for more of the day than he'd been smiling. Bedtimes were hard, mornings were hard – it was all really, really hard.

And honestly, I felt like a failure as a mum – why were the other kids bounding in with smiles on their faces? Where had I gone wrong?

I'd get in my car after drop-off ready for my commute to work and would crumble in tears. This became so frequent that I started to wait until after drop-off to put my mascara on because I knew it would soon be smudged by my tears. I felt lost and unsupported, and I just didn't know what to do.

That's why my jaw hit the floor the moment the school uttered those words. Have you ever been in one of those situations where someone says something and you just can't respond because you're in so much shock? And then about an hour later you come up with a million incredible responses, but it's too late?! Well, this was one of those situations.

Just to set the scene here, I'm no wallflower – my friends would describe me as strong, confident and more than capable of standing my ground – but, as I'm sure you can relate, dealing with things around your kids can bring even the strongest of people to their knees!

At the time, I was working as a senior Global HR Director in a FTSE 100 company. I was responsible for working with CEOs of large organisations with 60,000 or more people to support their teams in building leadership and resilience. I was lucky to travel the world and work with universities like Harvard Business School to bring the latest science and research around emotional health, managing stress, change and building resilience into organisations. It was a pretty cool job and I'd worked very hard to get where I had, so I was not unfamiliar with dealing with difficult situations.

I tell you this because I want you to know that wherever you are on your journey right now, if you've ever felt weak at the knees or hugely vulnerable in dealing with a challenge with your child – you're definitely not alone! These are some of the toughest times as a parent and the fact that you may have experienced them makes you just as human as the next parent. I'm here to tell you that you're doing an amazing job, it will all be OK. I believe in you!

OK, I digress, back to the story.

I shuffled out of the school, got myself home, poured a glass of wine and started to make a plan. A plan to support my child who was struggling with the transition into school – it was clear from the school's response, or lack thereof, that I was going to be doing this on my own.

I really felt that it was nothing major, just some settling in wobbles, a little separation anxiety and a feeling of not necessarily 'fitting in' with the other children. But I knew that there was at risk of it escalating into more if I didn't intervene, which is why I'd sought help from the school.

As I sat down and lost myself in my thoughts, and that glass of wine(!), I started to map out all of the areas that I needed to support my child with:

* Managing his emotional responses when I wasn't there.
* Managing friendships with those who were different from him.
* Helping him to feel good about who he is so he has high self-esteem.

As I continued to jot down ideas, I had a realisation. Everything that I wanted to teach him was grounded in the exact research and science that I'd been teaching CEOs and their teams for the last 15 years! The only difference was that my child was four and I was used to teaching leaders who were forty plus!

I knew the science and I knew what my child needed, so I got to work.

For the next six months or so I dedicated myself (alongside a busy corporate job) to doing lots of work around developing my child's emotional regulation, resilience and self-esteem. I read over a hundred books, studied countless models and worked with lots of experts in the field. It was an intense but transformational time for me to be able to take all of that corporate knowledge and science and then apply it in the context of my child.

I learnt that there were so many competing theories and opinions but also that there is some very robust science and research about how to build resilience, self-esteem and mental well-being in children and, for that matter, in adults. I decided to only put into practice techniques that were validated in robust data and that I felt were a good fit for my family and circumstances.

The change in my son over these six months or so was so wonderful to watch. Don't get me wrong, he was, and remains, relatively quiet, but what changed was his ability to manage tough situations. He had some tools that he could use when I wasn't there, he seemed to be walking away from situations that were upsetting him and he was making friends.

His development was so noticeable that the school asked me what I'd done because they had seen this shift too. This time, I was ready with a response. I explained that I'd been focused on coaching him through a tough time and building his emotional toolkit.

I also enquired as to whether they'd heard of any of the experts or work I'd used as it had been so successful. They hadn't, and that's when I realised that a lot of teachers are not trained on how to deal with separation anxiety, low self-esteem or other low-level mental health issues.

I couldn't believe it. I was literally stunned. Not least because one of the things I had learnt through my own research was the importance of early intervention when it comes to mental health issues in children.

A note about teachers

Part of this research and learning journey really helped me to better understand the reality of what goes on in schools, specifically primary schools. I developed a deep respect for teachers and for the incredible work that they do.

I realised why those teachers in my child's school had reacted as they had. Sadly, the system in which we operate means that our curriculums and teacher training programmes are relatively static. This means that not all teachers are actually taught about building self-esteem and resilience in children. Their teacher training courses don't necessarily prepare them for situations like the one they were facing with my child. And so, in some cases, they just bring to the role whatever their 'view' of the right thing to do is, whether that's based in science or research, or what they experienced as a child.

The reality is that retraining all teachers to develop the level of knowledge and skills around building children's mental resilience and emotional well-being is just not tenable. While I fully believe this would be an investment that would pay back huge dividends, I now understand that this is just a by-product of the system, not the people themselves.

With hindsight, I'm grateful for the school's response because it put me on the path to discovering what actually works when it comes to building resilience and happiness. Had the school placated me or if I'd have let it 'sort itself out', who knows where my child and I would be now.

Let's look at the facts around mental health in our young people. This data is based on the UK, but, as we look around the developed world, there are similar trends and parallels:

* Half of all mental health problems manifest by the age of 14, with 75 per cent by the age of 24.[1]
* 1 in 3 adult mental health conditions relate directly to adverse childhood experiences.[2]

The case for teaching preventative skills to children is clearly there, but teachers simply aren't trained to support low-level issues around separation anxiety and self-esteem. Given the mental health crisis we face as a society, how can this be so?

This is no way me bashing teachers – they're some of the most wonderful people in our society – and I don't want you to feel that I don't understand or appreciate the incredible work teachers do day in and day out to support children's learning. I do. I also see how stretched they are and how under-resourced and under-funded schools are. I think one of the consequences of this is that they can't always step up to support a child like mine to the extent to which as parents we'd hope they could.

It was baffling to me that the statistics were showing this consistent increase in the incidence of mental health issues, but we were still largely focused on reacting versus preventing. For example, if a child is presenting with a diagnosable mental health issue there is an established system in place in the UK for them to be referred by the school to the CAMHS (Child and Adolescent Mental Health Services). The process is clear for schools, *if* a child is really struggling.

However, when the issue is low-level or in the very early stages, as was the case with my son, there is very little, if anything, in place. As a society, we wait to act until a child is so bad that they need a specialist – this seems a little crazy to me.

There is a famous saying: 'The definition of insanity is doing the same thing over and over and expecting different results.' Why, then, are we as a society still focusing mostly on reacting rather than preventing? Why are we still using an approach that is so out of sync with what is happening with our young people's mental health? Surely, we'll end up with the same result that we've been getting when it comes to mental ill health in our young people? Surely that's insane?

Our education system talks a lot about how to keep our bodies healthy through drinking water, healthy eating and taking regular exercise, but where is the conversation about mental health? Where is the proactivity to ensure that we understand what our brains need to stay healthy and happy too?

I'm not talking about mental health awareness here because the noise on that has been getting louder for a number of years, helped along by numerous celebrities speaking out on the issue. While this is really important and has a role to play, I am actually talking about something else. Yes, our awareness of mental health issues is definitely greater than it was a decade ago, but what about our awareness of solutions?

Most of the stories you read are about the problems or about how you can come back from having a mental health issue. I want to change this conversation so that we talk as much about proactive solutions and prevention as we do about reacting to an issue. For children, this is particularly important because if we want to truly reverse the mental health epidemic, we have to look at prevention as well as cure.

Sadly, a focus on prevention and teaching strategies to look after our mental health and our minds is just not as mainstream as it needs to be. That, though, is the focus of this book.

The myHappymind system

Just a few weeks after my meeting with the school, I was back into my usual crazy routine of work and parenting. I was just about to pack my bag for a flight the next day when I received a phone call which felt like a double-decker bus had crashed into me at a hundred miles an hour.

The call was to tell me that someone close to me had been sectioned under the Mental Health Act. Now, before you jump to any conclusions about their past (I know I would have done!), they had no history of mental ill health. In fact, on paper they had it all: a great job, a great family, nice holidays. But the pressure had all become too much and they'd simply burnt out under the stress of it all. I have since learnt that this can happen to any of us.

Visiting them in the secure mental hospital was one of the most traumatic experiences of my life; you'll know why if you've ever been to one. To see this person who I love so dearly be so poorly and so far removed from their normal self was just heartbreaking. It showed me how serious mental health issues can become if we don't address them early. As I drove back home late that night, I realised something: if mental health issues can affect my child who has grown up in a happy and loving home, and they can affect this person too, then they can affect anyone.

I decided there and then that I wanted to be part of the solution. I wanted to try to shift the culture in primary schools so that children were learning skills around looking after their own mental and emotional resilience from as young as possible.

When I got home, I told my husband I'd be quitting my job to start myHappymind – an organisation that would be dedicated to building resilience, self-esteem and, ultimately, well-being habits in primary school children. I wanted to do something to help fix the massive epidemic we face around mental health in our young people.

There is a famous saying: 'It always seems impossible until it's done.' I use this quote to share some of what was going on in my mind when I told my friends and family that this was what I was going to do, because I was faced with comments such as:

★ 'Have you lost your mind?' (Ironic I know!)
★ 'You have an amazing career.'
★ 'But you're not a teacher.'
★ 'You've never worked in schools.'
★ [Insert any number of other reasons why I can't!]

And all I kept thinking was this: many people have done far more extraordinarily difficult things than this, so I won't let the naysayers stop me. It did seem impossible at the beginning for sure, but I wasn't going to let anyone talk me out of pursuing this passion. In fact, my internal dialogue became: 'I can and I will; watch me!'

I quit my corporate job, leaving behind a very nice salary and a lot of perks, and I got to work. I spent six long months researching and talking to experts, and was then ready to launch an early version of our programme into primary schools.

It quickly accelerated from there as the feedback from schools was so positive. Fast forward to today and we're now proudly impacting hundreds of thousands of children through our NHS-backed programmes in schools, nurseries, homes and organisations – it's been a journey, but one that I am so proud of.

I use the word 'journey' because there have been moments throughout it which I could have never predicted – both good and bad! The growth of myHappymind has definitely not followed a straight line; I prefer to describe it as a squiggly one with lots of switchback turns, but always orienting upwards!

I am lucky to have parents and to have had an education that constantly reminded me that I can do anything I want to, as long as I'm kind and I work hard. In her book, *Everything is Figureoutable*, Marie Forleo said: 'Nothing in life is that complicated. You can do whatever you set your mind to if you just roll up your sleeves, get in there, and do it.' I couldn't agree more.

There's been a lot of self-growth too! It turns out that those big senior corporate jobs are very different (and much easier!) than starting and running your own business. But would I ever go back? No chance.

To serve and impact others through this work is the best thing I have ever done. When I started, it was all about helping my child and I had no intention of it growing into what it has become today. While I'm immensely proud of the impact we've created, my proudest moment remains seeing my child continue to cope with the ups and downs of life with the tools he's learnt.

The research- and science-based approach that I've taken has led me to develop a simple but powerful model which we apply in all of our programmes. This approach is called the 'myHappymind system', and I'm so excited to walk you through it in this book.

It's an absolute pleasure for me to be able to share this work with you so that you too can use it to positively impact your family.

Because you can, and you will, and I'm going to help you.

Let's get started.

Introduction

One of the things I noticed when I started to better understand the science of happiness was how many competing perspectives exist.

There are hundreds, if not thousands, of books on the topic and oh so many different opinions. Add to that the sometimes very strong views that we hear from friends, parents and in-laws and it's no wonder that we can end up feeling totally overwhelmed! So overwhelmed, in fact, that we get stuck and are unable to really move forward.

Overwhelm plays out in many elements of our day-to-day lives and often comes when we've invited so much into our lives that we just can't digest it. We may in fact be very motivated to learn and act, but the lack of a clear path makes us feel paralysed and anxious. There are so many options that we just don't know which to take and so we don't take any.

This is exactly where I found myself as I started to read books and listen to podcasts on how to improve my child's resilience and self-esteem. There were so many different perspectives and opinions that I was totally and utterly overwhelmed.

★ How on earth was I supposed to decide what to try?
★ How would I know what would work for my child?
★ How the heck could I get started?

Any of this sound familiar?!

One of the greatest joys for me in bringing you this book is the knowledge that you won't have to go through the same overwhelm that I did, because I've done the 'sifting through' bit for you. I've compiled strategies that are based on the latest research around happiness and well-being so you can get started right away.

All of the research has been boiled down into the award-winning simple but powerful myHappymind system used by hundreds of thousands of children and adults and the NHS across schools, nurseries, organisations and homes. My mission is to bring it to you in an approachable and digestible way so that you understand it as much as you need to, but so that you don't become overwhelmed by it.

I'll teach you the science behind how this all works, and I'll take you on a journey to understand why each part of the myHappymind system is so critical to building your child's mental well-being, resilience and happiness as well as equipping you with practical strategies that work for the whole family. No more overwhelm or fluff; just real, science-backed techniques that you can start using right away. Sound good?

The system is based on understanding, and applying what the science tells us really matters when it comes to building resilience, self-esteem and ultimately happiness, not only in children but in adults too. We shouldn't underestimate just how much of an impact our happiness and well-being as parents influences that of our children. We need to make sure that we, as parents, are OK before we look after our children or those others around us. Looking after ourselves is perhaps one of the hardest things as parents. From the moment those little cherubs come into this world, we become conditioned to look after their needs before our own. We wake up in the night compromising our own sleep to make sure they're OK and fed. We give up careers and jobs to be at home with them in those early months. We lose our social life for a while to make sure they feel secure and loved. We put them before us.

Despite knowing that we can only be our best self if we put our own health first, we rarely do. Yet, all of the time we're at risk of diminishing our own well-being in order to love and protect our children. It is an instinct and a power that is incredibly hard to resist, and most of us don't win the fight. I believe that most parents at some point hit a wall and say, 'It is just all too much, I need to get a bit of me back!' Have you ever felt like that? I know I have.

That's why we look at strategies for you as an adult as well as strategies for your child. As you work through each part of the myHappymind system, you'll develop a holistic view of how to positively impact your whole family's well-being. But, more than that, you'll finish the book with a clear plan on how to embed powerful yet practical habits and rituals for you and your child.

The Five Elements of the myHappymind System

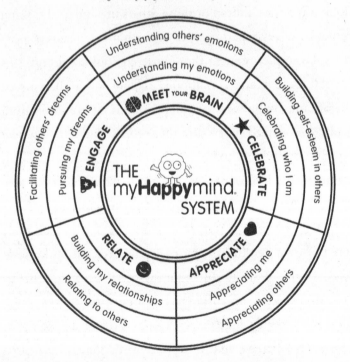

Introduction

Each of the chapters that follow delves into a different part of the myHappymind system. We'll take a look at the science and research behind each area, the role these factors play in society today and, finally, what you can do practically to develop yourself and support your child in this area.

One of the critical things to remember about this framework is that each part builds on the next, so the first part of the system is complemented by the second, and so on. It all hangs together, but by looking at each part separately you'll develop a depth of understanding that allows you to act on it.

Meet your brain

The first element of the myHappymind system is called 'Meet Your Brain'. Understanding how our brains work is absolutely critical in learning how to manage big emotions and deal with anxiety and stress. How on earth are we supposed to be able to support and manage these things if we don't really understand what's going on up there?

By the end of this chapter you'll not only have a really strong, working understanding of how our brains work alongside our emotions, you'll also have some practical strategies to start using right away. I'm also offering you some wonderful free digital resources that you can use too (see page 235 for details on how to access these).

So often it's in the moments in which our child is struggling the most that knowledge of what is happening in their brain is so critical. When I started to learn what was actually happening in my child's brain during a moment of panic or anxiety, everything changed for me. After learning what you will in this chapter, the parents I work with often say to me 'I just wish I'd understood this sooner' – I hope you'll have the same 'Aha!' moment!

Celebrate

The second component of the framework is called 'Celebrate' and it talks about one of the most powerful things I've ever learnt about humans and happiness. I know this sounds dramatic, but it's true!

In this chapter you'll learn exactly what it is that makes humans happy and, specifically, what builds our self-esteem. This may well come as a surprise to you – it definitely did to me!

Most of the time in organisations, schools or homes the focus of praise is around competence or what we've achieved. As parents, we'll often find ourselves celebrating our child's neat colouring, or getting picked for the A team, or getting 10/10 in a spelling test. These are all competence-based activities – they rely on our ability to do something. If you work in an organisation, you'll be familiar with performance reviews or being rewarded for what you have achieved and, once again, these are things that rely on our competence in a particular area.

As humans we learn that competence is what matters because it is competence that leads to praise. We also learn that praise equals love and self-worth. But, here's the thing – praising your child's competence or ability does not build their self-esteem!

In this chapter, I'll explain how you *do* build self-esteem and how with some very simple shifts you can start applying this knowledge right away. It has been one of the most eye-opening parts of my journey and I can't wait to share it with you.

Appreciate

The third component of the myHappymind system is called 'Appreciate'. As you've probably guessed, this is all focused around gratitude. We'll explore what true gratitude is and why it's so important to our happiness. If you're thinking 'My children have great manners, I've got this one down', that's wonderful; who doesn't love a polite child?! But that's not what we're talking about here. True gratitude looks quite different to remembering our Ps and Qs.

In this chapter you may find yourself highly surprised at the effect that gratitude has on our brains and our overall well-being and happiness. Think about a time when someone expressed real, deep gratitude to you. Maybe it was a friend expressing thanks for having supported them through a tough time. Or maybe you expressed gratitude to your child for tidying up their bedroom. Close your eyes for a minute and take yourself back to that moment when someone expressed gratitude to you – how did it feel? And what about when you've done something for someone else and they've not expressed gratitude? I'm willing to bet that felt less good. Am I right?

In this part of the myHappymind system, we'll be diving into why gratitude is so powerful and why it can evoke such strong emotions (both positively and negatively). We'll then explore some practical tools that you can use to get your child started with their very own gratitude habit.

Relate

Next up is 'Relate', which is all about understanding how to develop and maintain healthy relationships. I believe that this is one of the most challenging areas of parenting today. The way in which children build and maintain relationships has undoubtedly changed. The use of technology, especially as they grow older, sees them developing relationships through apps and games. Not only this, the way we as adults use technology is modelling a different approach to our children too.

We know from the science that positive relationships are one of the most fundamental components of our happiness. But do we really know how to ensure that we and our children build and maintain positive ones?

As much as we can wrap children up when they are little and protect them from the child who is being unkind in the soft play centre, we can't negotiate these things for them forever. Once they start school, they need the skills to build and maintain positive relationships on their own. We can't always be there for them, but we can give them the skills to manage when they're on their own.

This part of the system looks at how we can build and maintain positive relationships and help our children to do the same.

Engage

The final element of the myHappymind system is 'Engage' and it's all about how we can encourage children to engage in the world through positive achievement.

One of the most powerful ways to impact our happiness is through the accomplishment of goals, through making things happen or getting things done. And, of course, much of our lives are structured around this.

At school, children get set homework and at work we have objectives. If we are a stay-at-home parent, making sure that our children's seemingly endless needs are met – whether that's emotionally, educationally or otherwise – gives us our own to-do list! But these 'to-do list goals' that are set by others or by our circumstances are not what I'm talking about here. While they are, of course, important, they don't really contribute to our well-being.

This part of the framework is about exploring which types of goals are important to our happiness and how we can encourage children to set and strive for them.

You are the expert in your own child

There's no such thing as a one-size-fits-all approach when it come to your child's well-being. This book doesn't contain a 'do this and you'll make your child happy' golden ticket (sorry!). However, it does provide you with a practical guide to the factors that have the most impact on self-esteem and well-being.

In giving you this full picture, you can then take your pick of the areas that you think are going to be most impactful for your child. Don't worry – I'll guide you through this process.

But, here's the truth . . . no one knows your child better than you. No one has your incredible parental gut instinct that will tell you what they need. Even if you're not feeling in tune with that right now, I will help you to tune back in.

Yes, there are lots of experts out there, many of whom you may have already seen or talked to, but they will never know your child as intimately as you do. Parental instinct is a particularly powerful tool and it should never be ignored.

I remember hearing advice when I was on my journey that I just knew wouldn't work for my child. Was I a doctor? No. Did I consider myself an expert at that point? No. Was I certain that the strategies being advised would make my child feel angry and stressed? Yes.

Introduction

What I was then, and what I remain today, is an expert on my child and I knew that certain strategies just wouldn't work. Everything changed for me once I knew the science because I understood all of the options that I had. Once I appreciated the full 'list' of strategies that I could use, I was able to design a menu that worked for us as a family. Think of this book like your very own a la carte menu – you'll need to see exactly what's on the menu before you decide what you want to choose, but there's something for everyone!

Never ignore your parental gut instinct. It's an absolute superpower and one that we should all use.

How to Use This Book

Before we get started, I want to share a few pieces of advice on how best to use this book. You've invested the time and money into it, so let's really make it count.

Don't get in your own way

> 'There are plenty of difficult obstacles in your path.
> Don't allow yourself to be one of them.'
> **Ralph Marston - Greatday.com**

So often the stories that we tell ourselves stop us from moving forward. Sometimes, we're not even aware of these stories because they're being told so deeply in our subconscious mind. Stories such as:

* 'I already know this – I heard it on a TED Talk once.'
* 'My child will never respond to this, they just aren't built like that.'
* 'I'm just not cut out to be *that* kind of parent.'

The one thing that all of these stories have in common is that they are unhelpful and untrue. When you feel these thoughts popping up, I want you to try to catch them. Catch them, and then flip them on their head so that they become positive questions or statements. This might feel tricky at first but, the more you do it, the easier it'll get and it will transform your learning experience.

For example, rather than: 'I already know this – I heard it on a TED Talk once', flip it into: 'I am familiar with this. How can I take my understanding even deeper?'

Instead of: 'My child will never respond to this, they just aren't built like that', flip it into: 'This feels different to what I've tried before. I am willing to explore something new.'

And flip 'I am just not cut out to be *that* kind of parent' into: 'This isn't something that I currently do, but I am open to trying a new approach.'

Introduction

Do the work

'If anything is worth doing, do it with all your heart.'
Buddha

Each part of the system comes with some reflection exercises and these are really important, so please don't be tempted to skip them!

I get it – you're busy, you feel like you've got the gist of the chapter and you just want to start the next one and, honestly, I've done that with other books too. But here's the thing, you'll get so much more value out of this book if you trust my process and do the reflection exercises. Because, actually, it's more than a book; it's also a mini-course that, if used as I have intended, will allow you to not only learn, but also to reflect and plan your action steps.

There are a couple of reasons why these reflection exercises are so important:

1. Our brains process information in a totally different and more permanent way when we write things down.
2. We often don't fully understand how we feel about a situation until we've reflected on it and written it down.

For these reasons, it will be incredibly powerful for you to take a few seconds to complete the exercises.

Deal? OK, good. Now that we're agreed on that, make sure you've always got a pen handy so that you can scribble some notes down as we go through each chapter, or turn to the 'Lovely Notes' section on pages 231–34 and jot down your thoughts as you go along.

Don't dip in and out

> *'Stay committed to your decisions,*
> *but flexible in your approach.'*
> **Tony Robbins, *Awaken the Giant Within***

I know how it goes – you've bought the book, you read the first chapter and then, life happens! You leave it on your bedside table, Netflix calls and, well, it takes you a while to get back into your reading habit.

Here's a tip for you – try to dedicate some proper time to read this book so that you read it all in a relatively short period of time. This way you'll ensure that you take it all in.

I recommend that you read the book all the way through before you move into full implementation. This will give you the complete picture and help you to really get underneath the meaning of each area. Then, once you have that full overview, you can come back to it and read more about each section again as you need to. There is a very intentional order in terms of the chapters, but once you've got the whole picture you can dive into particular chapters whenever you need to.

Introduction

Comparisonitis is a disease – don't catch it

'Comparison is the thief of joy.'
President Theodore Roosevelt

OK, so here is your first dose of tough love! I firmly believe that becoming a parent opens up some of the most joyous moments of our lives. I also think that it is one of the times in our lives when we are most likely to compare ourselves with others. We start right at the beginning with thoughts and conversations with other parents like:

* 'How many times do they wake up through the night?'
* 'How many spoonfuls of mashed-up carrot did they have for lunch?'
* 'Oh, you're not breastfeeding?'
* 'They walked when they were how old?'
* 'Oh . . . you give them pre-made baby food!'
* 'Have you left them for a night yet with someone else?'
* 'Are you going back to work?'

And so it continues . . . And while many of these questions are well-meaning, they inevitably cause us to compare ourselves. And while some of this is natural, some of it is unhealthy.

It can lead us to catch 'comparison-itis', a disease of our thoughts whereby we measure our own progress or that of our children against other people. We measure it against our friend or that person we follow on Instagram who just seems to have it so 'together'.

This can lead to thoughts like:

* 'How is their house always so tidy?' (It's not by the way – they just tidied it up to take that photo.)
* 'Their child never seems to look sad.' (They have their moments, they just don't photograph them for Instagram!)
* 'They just look so together as a mum.' (I am willing to bet that they ugly-cry sometimes too!)

My point here is this: the only thing that I want you to measure your progress against when it comes to your child's resilience, self-confidence and happiness is where they were yesterday. No one else's journey is relevant. The only thing that matters is that you make baby steps forward each and every day.

When we start to compare ourselves, we can get lost in a spiral of feeling like we're not doing enough, saying enough, preparing enough, *being* enough! And does any of this actually help us move forward? No – the irony is that by comparing ourselves we end up going backwards. It makes us feel so down on ourselves that we can sink into overwhelm and take no action.

And so *please* avoid comparing yourself to others, just focus on you and your family.

Introduction

Be kind to yourself

'I talk to myself the way I would talk to someone I really love.'
Brené Brown

Finally, I want you to be gentle with yourself as you go through this book. It's intended to open your eyes to some new options and approaches. It is not intended to tell you that what you're doing now is wrong or that you have to change.

Remember the a la carte menu analogy that I used earlier? Keep that in mind – there will be things you learn that you think *yes*, that is what we need more of as a family. There may be other areas that you feel you're already covering, and that's great!

My intention is for you to feel you have some new strategies to try and that you have a total picture of all the options available to build your child's resilience and happiness.

The fact that you're here tells me so much about what an amazing parent you already are. You care enough to learn and reflect, and I know you're an action-taker because you bought this book. You've got this.

OK, are you ready? Let's dive in.

CHAPTER 1
Meet Your Brain

'If the human brain were so simple that we could
understand it, we would be so simple that we couldn't.'
Emerson M. Pugh

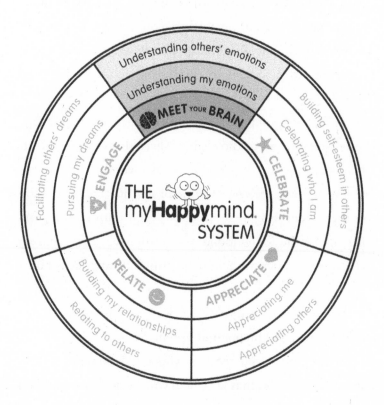

I'm going to start this chapter by acknowledging that there
is *so* much that the world's best neuroscientists still don't

know about the brain. I'd also like to make it plainly clear that I am not, nor do I pretend to be, a neuroscientist!

However, I do understand enough to give you a working understanding of the brain, particularly around our emotions and behaviours. My goal in this chapter is to help you to understand what is going on in the brain during periods of calm and during times of stress, because, with this knowledge, your whole perspective around managing yourself and supporting your child in times of worry will change. It will help you to develop your happy mind and to support your child in having a happy mind too.

Before we jump in, let's come back to the myHappymind system and acknowledge where this component sits relative to the rest of the areas we'll cover:

As you can see, 'Meet Your Brain' sits right at the top of the system. It's where all of our programmes start, and it really is the foundational piece from which everything else flows. Understanding your brain's behaviour is absolutely critical to understanding the rest of the factors that affect your well-being. Meet Your Brain is the backbone of the entire myHappymind system.

There are many reasons why developing an understanding of the brain is so critical when it comes to building a happy mind – from how we respond to children's emotions to how our thoughts impact our behaviours – and we'll explore these as we go through this chapter.

By the end of the chapter you will have a whole new insight into why we react as we do, particularly during times of stress and worry, and how we can shift our behaviours to transform how we experience the world. Let's get started.

How Does Our Brain Work?

'A mind is like a parachute.
It doesn't work if it is not open.'
Frank Zappa

We're going to spend some time understanding how our brains work. Now, don't panic, this isn't going to be a really detailed science lesson! But it is going to equip you with some key concepts which, in turn, will give you a working knowledge of the brain.

Then, we'll use your new-found knowledge about the brain to start to recognise why we respond in certain ways at certain times. After that, we'll do some reflection and action planning so that you can start to integrate this into how you approach moments of high stress with your child.

We're going to focus on looking at three key parts of the brain. Understanding these and how they interact together will really help you to start to see why your child reacts the way they do and how you can approach supporting them differently.

The hippocampus

The first part of the brain that we're going to learn about is the 'hippocampus'.

hip-*uh*-**kam**-p*uh*s

The hippocampus is where all of our memories get stored. I like to describe it as being like a huge scrapbook where everything that we learn and everything that we experience is kept.

Anything that you've ever learnt, any memory that you've ever had, will be in your hippocampus. The interesting thing about the hippocampus is that it stores the memory that we have, but it also stores the emotion that is associated with that memory. For example, I went to the park and I felt happy, or I had a meeting with my boss and I felt really nervous about it. Every memory we have is stored as both the event or what happened and the emotion or how we felt.

The amygdala

The second part of our brain is called the 'amygdala'.

uh-**mig**-d*uh*-l*uh*

The amygdala is the part of our brain whose only job is to keep us safe from danger. It spends all of its time scanning and then reacting to danger.

You may not have heard of the amygdala, but you have probably heard of the term 'fight, flight or freeze'. When the amygdala senses danger, it activates causing us to respond with either a fight, flight or freeze reaction, in order to keep us safe.

The prefrontal cortex

Finally, the 'prefrontal cortex' is the part of our brain that's responsible for logic and decision-making.

pree-**fruhn**-tl **kawr**-teks

The prefrontal cortex analyses situations and helps us to use logic to decide what we're going to do.

Because many of our programmes are taught to children, we've created a character – 'Team HAP' – to help them to remember these three parts of the brain. In my experience, this character has also helped our adult students to remember them too, so I've included it below for you:

As you can see, Team HAP has three heads(!), each symbolising a different part of the brain: H for hippocampus, A for amygdala and P for prefrontal cortex. This is a character that you're going to get to know and love. Children tend to respond really well to visual cues like this, so this should help you no end when you start working with your child (I've included a fun printable for you in the digital resources – see page 235).

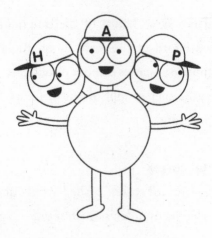

As with all teams, Team HAP works best when all the elements are working together – when information can pass between the hippocampus, the amygdala and the prefrontal cortex, we can perform at our best.

For example, when we can recall memories (hippocampus) and make logical decisions (prefrontal cortex), and when we analyse if a situation is dangerous or not (amygdala) and act accordingly, then we can be our best self.

However, the reality is that sometimes Team HAP works well together and sometimes it doesn't. Let's explore why this happens and what the consequences are through the lens of two different scenarios.

Scenario 1: We feel happy, safe and calm

In this scenario, all three elements of Team HAP are smiling, they are talking to each other and all parts of the brain are active. As a result, information is flowing freely between the three parts of the brain. In these situations, we can make good decisions, recall memories and keep ourselves safe, and so we can be the best version of ourselves. This is where we want our brain, and our child's brain, to be for as much of the time as possible.

Scenario 2: We feel stressed, worried or sad

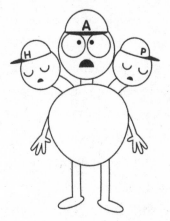

Let's take a look at what happens when we feel worried, stressed or sad. As you can see, something has changed – the amygdala, which is the slightly worried looking guy in the middle, has taken control of the brain. It's done this because it's detected danger and so has become activated.

The amygdala has reacted to keep us safe from this danger and in that process our hippocampus, which is where all of our memories are stored, and our prefrontal cortex, which is where our decision-making happens, have shut down or gone to sleep. We'll learn more about why this happens later on.

Now that the hippocampus and prefrontal cortex have gone to sleep, we can no longer access our memories or make logical decisions. So in situations where the amygdala has reacted in response to danger, the only part of our brain which is active is the amygdala. This means that the only response available to us is to fight, flight or freeze.

Let's look at a couple of examples to further understand the impact of the amygdala taking control and shutting down the hippocampus and prefrontal cortex.

Your child has a spelling test and they've worked hard for it but, for whatever reason, they really worry about spelling tests. Because of this worry, the minute the teacher says it's time for the test, their amygdala detects danger and activates, and then the hippocampus (memory) and prefrontal cortex (decision-making) go to sleep.

As soon as the hippocampus goes to sleep all of that revision they've done for the test is effectively useless because they can't access those memories. The prefrontal cortex has also gone to sleep and so they can't make a logical choice about how to respond. The only response available to them is therefore to fight, flight or freeze. This might result in them getting upset or angry about the test (fighting), wanting to leave the classroom (fleeing) or just sitting there not knowing what to do (freezing).

Let's take another example using an adult who has a job interview. They are desperate to land this job and have done hours of preparation to ensure they come across well and get in all of the experiences that make them the perfect candidate. They walk into the interview room, see that there are three interviewers waiting to greet them and just panic. Their amygdala activates because they interpret this situation as danger. Again, in that process their hippocampus (memories) will close down as will their prefrontal cortex (decision-making).

All of those incredible experiences that they've had are lost in their hippocampus and they forget to mention them. All of the preparation that they've done the night before just goes out of the window and they don't perform anywhere near as well as they could have done had they been able to remain calm.

You may have read both of these examples and thought they don't apply to you or your child. However, there will be some situations which do cause your amygdala to react. Is it the wasp in the beer garden in the summer? Your annual performance meeting with your boss? Confrontation with a family member? For your child it might be when they are asked to stand up in assembly and share something or maybe when they meet a new group of people or join a new club.

We all have different situations that cause our amygdala to activate. What is the same for all of us, though, is how this impacts Team HAP. When the amygdala activates, the hippocampus and prefrontal cortex go to sleep in all of us.

To help you to ground this in examples that are real for you, I'd like you to note down the situations that cause your amygdala to react and then those that that cause your child's to react too.

What causes your amygdala to react?

....

....

....

What causes your child's amygdala to react?

....

....

....

The Amygdala: Our Best Friend and Our Worst Enemy!

The amygdala is often referred to as the reptilian brain because it's remarkably similar in function to that of a reptile. Yes, our amygdala responds in exactly the same way as a crocodile's! Because the amygdala hasn't evolved much at all since we humans lived in caves, it's not a particularly sophisticated part of the brain. While it's incredible at reacting, it does not have the ability to analyse, so it cannot tell whether a danger or threat is real (such as a sabre-toothed tiger approaching) or perceived (such as standing onstage and delivering a speech).

When we were cave-dwellers this was incredibly helpful as it meant that we could quickly react to real physical danger and stay alive. When the danger is a real threat to our physical safety, the amygdala could be described as our best friend because it will cause us to respond by either fighting, fleeing or freezing. Ultimately, it will save our life!

For example, imagine you are in a bar and a fight breaks out near you. It's your amygdala that will quickly react forcing you to fight, flight or freeze thereby keeping you safe in this situation.

However, the problem with the amygdala is that, because it cannot analyse and tell if a danger is real or perceived, if we think something is dangerous (whether it is or not), the amygdala reacts. So it reacts to a real danger such as the bar fight or a perceived danger such as public speaking in just the same way – by fighting, fleeing or freezing.

This is why I like to describe the amygdala as being our best friend when the danger is real and our worst enemy when the danger is perceived. When the danger is real, we want our amygdala to do its job. But when the danger isn't real and the amygdala reacts, it is incredibly helpful to learn how to calm it down. Take a look at your reflections from earlier as to when this happens for you and your child. It is in these moments that we wish we could control our amygdala more. The good news is that we can!

Before we dive into the strategies to help calm the amygdala down, let's learn a little bit more about what actually happens when the amygdala is activated.

What happens when our amygdala reacts?

When our amygdala senses danger and reacts, all of the oxygen floods from our brain into our arms, legs and torso – ready to fight, flight or freeze. During this process, the hippocampus and prefrontal cortex go to sleep due to the lack of oxygen in the brain. This happens exceptionally fast as the amygdala is so finely tuned and incredibly effective.

Remember, our amygdala will respond in this way, whether the danger is real or perceived, because it thinks it is saving our life. When the danger is real we don't want it to stop doing its thing! We want it to respond by either fighting, fleeing or freezing to keep us safe. However, we do want to be able to calm the amygdala down when the danger is perceived or reacting to something that we just think is dangerous, e.g. that spelling test.

Let's take an example of a person whose amygdala reacts when they have to give a speech. Picture the scene: they've been asked to be best man and the time has come to give the much-anticipated best man's speech.

For whatever reason, they perceive public speaking as a danger and so, as the time to give the speech approaches, they start to sense danger and their amygdala activates. When this happens, the oxygen floods to the body so that it has as much energy as possible to fight, flight or freeze in response to this perceived danger. In that process, the hippocampus (memories) and prefrontal cortex (decision-making) shut down.

So the best man is stood there, in front of the wedding guests and their best friend who is hoping the speech isn't too inappropriate . . . and they just freeze. They cannot recall the speech they've memorised because their hippocampus is asleep, and they cannot take logical steps to calm themselves down because the prefrontal cortex is asleep too.

So, what happens?

Well, they'll appear rather flustered and stressed and will probably mumble through those words that they spent so long preparing and then sit down as fast as they can. The rest of their day, and beyond, will be filled with regret and thoughts of 'What on earth happened?!' and 'Why couldn't I just pull myself together?!'

What might be an alternative in this situation if we're the speech-giver and we know that this might happen? The only way that we can move out of this amygdala-controlled state is to wake up the hippocampus and the prefrontal cortex.

Remember that they went to sleep in the first place because they were starved of oxygen because it had all flooded to the arms and legs and torso. Therefore, to wake them up again we need to get oxygen back up to the brain so that the hippocampus and prefrontal cortex can start to work again.

By waking them up they can start to play their role in helping us to make logical decisions and to recall our memories. This is a technique that I like to call 'happy breathing'. This is grounded in similar science as mindfulness or meditation, but we've found that by naming it happy breathing it gets more traction with children (and adults!). Essentially, it's all about getting oxygen back up to the brain by taking slow, deep breaths.

What might have happened for the best man if he'd been able to do some happy breathing before his speech? If he knew about this technique, he could have used it just as he started to feel the amygdala taking hold. As a result of this he wouldn't have forgotten his words because the hippocampus would still be awake and his prefrontal cortex would have helped him to just get through the speech and do a fabulous job. You can see how different these scenarios are, just from this small difference in his approach. Isn't it amazing how powerful our breath can be?

Happy Breathing

I'd like you to try this happy breathing exercise right now so that you can start to see how calming the breath can be for your body and mind. There's also an audio-based happy breathing exercise in the free digital resources to use with your child (see page 235). If you've never done any kind of breathing work like this before, please don't worry – I promise it is really simple and really powerful!

We're going to do an exercise that I call 'finger breathing' and, once you've read the instructions below, I'd like you to put the book down and have a go.

All you're going to do is hold out a hand in front of you with your fingers spread out wide – it doesn't matter which hand you choose.

Next, use the index finger of your other hand to gently trace up and down your fingers. As you go down one finger you'll breathe out and as you trace up the next finger, you'll breathe in.

Got it? The following diagram should help:

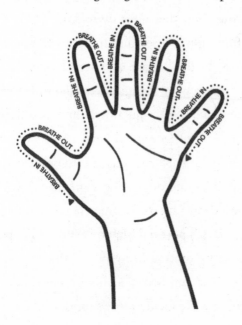

Now, put the book down and, closing your eyes, trace your entire hand 10 times. When you've done this, just take a moment to notice how you feel before you open your eyes and pick up the book again.

OK, welcome back! How did that feel? Write down three words to describe how you feel now. And if you didn't do the exercise . . . come on, go back and give it a try!

....

....

....

What you just did during that happy breathing session was really focus on your breathing and send lots of oxygen up to your brain. Whether your amygdala was activated or not, hopefully you can see that this helped you to relax. If you were to do this before an event like the best man's speech you'd stop your amygdala taking full control, your hippocampus wouldn't shut down and you'd remember those magical words you'd planned!

This particular happy breathing exercise is clever because, by focusing our mind on tracing our fingers, we're able to take our mind off any distracting thoughts and just focus on our breath. It's particularly powerful and popular with children because of its sensory focus – they really enjoy it.

Happy breathing is a great tool to introduce to your child when they are facing those situations that aren't real, but that cause their amygdala to react. Whether that is swimming lessons, or tests, or whatever it might be! However, it's important to note that introducing any new technique to a child can take some time and, of course, all children will go at their own pace – your child may take to it immediately or they may take a little longer to get the hang of it. Either way stick with it because it will pay dividends once they start recognising that they can use happy breathing to calm their amygdala during times of worry or stress.

When introducing this technique to your child for the first time, I'd suggest doing so when they are feeling calm and happy – such as bedtime – and simply explain that it helps us to relax our minds. We will work up to them being able to use it when they are feeling distressed, but we have to get them familiar with it first. In fact, if we try to introduce this technique when they're feeling distressed it can backfire because they aren't ready to receive this kind of logic-based strategy. The key is to get your child used to this technique while all the elements of Team HAP are wide awake. Once you feel that your child is comfortable and has really got the hang of it, then it's time to explain that this technique can be used when they start to feel those wobbles or begin to feel upset.

I'd like to share a story here which illustrates how my son uses this technique on autopilot now having practised it for some time. When he started in Year 4 (some years after first learning this technique) it was his first day of school and the teacher announced that she wanted all of the children to introduce themselves and say three things about their summer holiday. This is the type of situation which, at the time, was my son's worst nightmare – public speaking was one of the areas that caused his amygdala to react. He knew this, though, and so as soon as he heard that he would need to stand up he started to do his finger breathing under the desk, to calm himself down before his turn.

To his teacher it looked like he was just fidgeting with something under his desk and so she asked him, 'What are you playing with under your desk?' He replied, 'I'm not playing with anything – I am doing my happy breathing.'

'What is that?' the teacher asked.

'Well, when I am feeling nervous my amygdala reacts and it sends my hippocampus and prefrontal cortex to sleep which means that I can't remember things. Happy breathing stops this from happening.'

Let's just say she was a little surprised and later called me to tell me how impressed she was that he knew all of this *and* had a strategy to cope with a tricky situation. This is not something teachers see every day, but it is incredible to think that you can and will equip your child with these types of coping strategies if you stick with it and create this habit.

Let's now spend some time reflecting on when happy breathing might be most useful for both you and your child. Hopefully, you can start to see how having a technique like this in your toolkit to teach your child is really useful. Look back at page 28 to see when your child's amygdala reacts, but the danger isn't real. One of the most common 'Aha!' moments that the parents I work with have is based around this knowledge of what's happening for their child when the amygdala is activated but the danger isn't real.

Happy breathing and dopamine

I want to spend some time talking about the other positive effects of happy breathing. These extend far beyond better managing moments of panic and worry as we've just explored.

When we do happy breathing, the feel-good hormone dopamine gets released in our brain. This is the same hormone that gets released when we laugh or have fun with our friends. It makes us feel happy, positive and at ease in the moment and, over the long term, can help us to manage our stress levels. This is because it has the effect of counteracting the stress hormones in our brain. The more dopamine we have in our brain, the lower our stress levels over time – sounds good, right?

Dopamine is also addictive to the brain, so when we do an activity that releases dopamine, our brains are encouraged to do that activity again and again. This is why establishing a regular habit of happy breathing is so good for us. As well as helping us through tough moments where our amygdala may have reacted, happy breathing has a long-term well-being effect too. By getting into a regular habit of happy breathing, we're actually managing the levels of the stress hormone cortisol in the brain and therefore lowering worry and anxiety. Getting your child into the regular habit of happy breathing (at times of calm and at times of worry) will help them to have this regular flow of dopamine in their brains and, in turn, manage their stress levels. Consequently, they'll build their resilience skills and coping strategies, and will learn that they can face and overcome tough times with happy breathing. What a wonderful gift to be able to give your child.

Why Other Strategies Don't Work

As parents we often respond to our children when their amygdala is in control or we see big negative emotions with one of two strategies. We're going to explore those strategies now with the use of an example. Let's take the child whose amygdala activates when it is time for their swimming lesson – they have a real fear of the water and, whenever it is time to get in, their amygdala reacts.

Logical thought and reasoning

Imagine your child is crying because they don't want to get in the water; they're saying they're scared and they won't get in the pool. In this situation, we might say something like: 'All you need to do is get in the swimming pool and do what the teacher says, and you'll be fine. Nothing bad will happen – the teacher is right there.'

With this approach you're trying to talk to their prefrontal cortex by using logic-based language but, remember, their amygdala is activated and so the prefrontal cortex is fast asleep. They simply cannot access that logical part of their brain because the amygdala is in control and so these words will have no impact. In fact, they may make them even more distressed. When your child is distressed and their amygdala is activated, trying to calm them down using logic is a waste of time.

Memory-based strategies

Now imagine that your child is continuing to get more upset. You've tried the logic-based strategy and that didn't work, so you try something else. Your child is lashing out, pulling their swimming cap off and refusing to get in the water and you say something like: 'Just relax, you were absolutely fine last time. Remember when you got out of the water at the end of the lesson? You had a great time!'

This is a memory-based strategy – you're trying to get them to remember that they've been here before and everything was absolutely fine. Guess which part of the brain you're trying to access here? Yep, that's right – the hippocampus, but this is also fast asleep because the amygdala is in control. So again, you're trying to access a part of the brain that is simply not available to your child at that point in time.

Parents will often say to me, 'Oh my goodness, this is me! I always try to use logic- or memory-based strategies when they are upset and now I see why that is a waste of time!' Can you take a moment to think about whether this applies to you?

What *can* you do in these moments?

Both memory- and logic-based strategies will work with your child, but only when all elements of Team HAP are awake. When the amygdala is activated and the hippocampus and prefrontal cortex are asleep, the child can't access those parts of the brain and so these strategies just won't work. The only thing that you can usefully do for your child (or yourself) when their amygdala has taken control and you know the danger isn't real is to try to wake up the hippocampus and the prefrontal cortex so that they can start recalling memories (about that last swimming lesson) and make good choices about how to respond. The only way to do this is with happy breathing. This will send oxygen back up to the brain allowing them to wake up Team HAP.

By simply focusing on their breathing you'll be able to help your child to calm down and move through these moments far more easily and with much less stress. Different techniques will work for different children, and so you'll likely need to experiment here. It could be sitting with them and stroking their head, or holding them tight, or leaving them to breathe quietly alone. You'll figure out what is best with some practice, but the key thing to remember is to calm them down first and, once all the elements of Team HAP are working well together again, you can start using memory-based strategies (because the hippocampus will be awake) and logic-based strategies (because the prefrontal cortex is awake). As parents, we need to learn to pick our moments and make sure we use the right strategies at the right time.

Once you have got the hang of happy breathing you'll see how transformational it can be. By putting all of your energy and focus into soothing your child rather than trying to 'fix' the problem in the moment, you'll get to a solution far sooner and everyone will be much calmer too!

I'm going to close this part of the chapter with a short but powerful story about one of my myHappymind parents:

This mum has a little boy who gets incredibly distressed and overwhelmed when he has homework that he finds difficult. Her approach in these situations used to be using logic with him and telling him to calm down and get on with it.

She would say things like: 'I know you can do this because you've done these sums before' or 'This isn't hard, you just need to remember what you did last time' or 'The sooner you start, the sooner you'll be finished and you can go and play on your Xbox.'

Guess what? None of these things helped and, if anything, he would become more distressed. When she learnt about Team HAP, she realised that he perceived difficult homework as a danger and so his amygdala was activating.

Once she realised that his hippocampus was asleep, so he couldn't remember having done this work before, and that his prefrontal cortex was also asleep, so he was struggling with logical thought, she changed her entire approach.

She started to do happy breathing with him before she would even mention homework so that she could use logic- and memory-based strategies to prepare him. She was doing this just before the amygdala had a chance to take hold and it totally transformed homework time!

Think about what you've learnt and reflect on how you can bring this into your everyday parenting. This is when you'll experience the most benefits from the myHappymind system – when you can take it from learning to action.

Let's take some time now to reflect. Are there any situations with your child when you could try to use this same strategy? Note down below when you think it might be most useful for your child:

....

....

....

What about for you? Could you use this strategy too?

....

....

....

Now that we have explored how the brain works and how we can manage it when it is reacting in an unhelpful way, we're going to take this knowledge to a deeper level and look at the role our minds play in our behaviour more broadly.

Our Thoughts and Behaviour

We're now going to explore the incredible power of our thoughts and specifically how they impact our behaviour. To do this we're going to look at the 'Thoughts à Feelings à Behaviour' model. It's an incredibly powerful way to see how what happens in our brains – our thoughts – directly impacts the actions we take, or our behaviour.

Used alongside your knowledge of the brain, it will help you to build perspective on how you can start to shift and manage those amygdala moments in your child and help them move through them with more ease.

This model describes the relationship between our thoughts, our feelings and our behaviour. It's remarkably simple yet incredibly powerful:

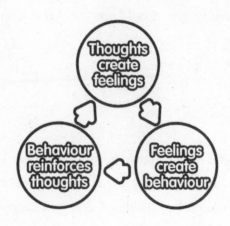

As you can see, right at the beginning of this cycle are our thoughts, which originate from our brains. Our thoughts, whether positive or negative, then lead us to feel certain emotions. If we're having positive thoughts, for example: 'This party is going to be so much fun', then we'll feel positive emotions such as excitement and happiness. Consequently, our behaviour will be positive too. We'll show up to the party in a good mood and contribute positively to the gathering. In this example our positive thoughts led to positive feelings which led to positive behaviour.

Guess what? The opposite is also true. If we are having negative thoughts about something, let's say a difficult conversation with a family member or our boss, we'll have negative feelings about it and then our behaviour will be negative too.

Let's now use the model to look at an example of a child facing a situation that they're concerned about. We'll use the swimming lesson example again (but you can insert any example here that your child worries about).

Let's start at the top of the Thoughts ➔ Feelings ➔ Behaviour model and consider what thoughts they may be having. They may be thinking things like:

★ 'What if I go underwater?'
★ 'What if I get water in my mouth?'
★ 'If I'm out of my depth, will anyone come and help me?'

The feelings that will follow these thoughts may be of fear, worry or even panic. Then comes the behaviour (as a result of the feelings). Maybe they'll cry, refuse to get into the pool or get angry. There could be any number of behaviours, but if the feelings were negative then the behaviours will be too.

How a child responds to negative thoughts will depend on their character and may differ based on the situation too. You'll know what your child's 'go-to' stress response is. The key point here is that their negative thoughts led to negative feelings and then negative behaviours. Now that you have this model in your toolkit, you can start to make a lasting impact on how your child deals with worrying situations.

You can see how critical a role our thoughts (which originate in our brains) play in our feelings or emotions and our consequent actions or behaviours. Henry Ford said, 'Whether you believe you can do a thing or not, you are right.' This quote sums up the power of our thoughts beautifully. They are so critical to how we feel, how we behave and, therefore, the results that we achieve. One of the most common 'Aha!' moments that the parents I coach have is when they realise how this model is playing out for them and for their children.

In almost 95 per cent of cases my students, who include CEOs, teachers and parents of three-year-olds (!), are not familiar with this model and its content. And why would they be? It's not taught in schools. It's not taught in organisations. So how are we supposed to know this? The good news is that now you do! And you can use it to your massive advantage both with yourself and with your child. Here's how . . .

When your child is experiencing negative thoughts and feelings, whether they are manifesting in tears, withdrawal or a full-blown meltdown, what you're seeing is the behaviour (the last part of this cycle). This behaviour is flowing from their negative feelings and their negative feelings are coming from their negative thoughts.

Many of us deal with these situations by only tackling the last part of this cycle – the behaviour that our child is showing us e.g. the tears, the backchat or the meltdown. Of course we do, because we're dealing with the thing that is right in front of our eyes. But what if I told you that just responding to the behaviour is a bit like putting an old plaster on a leaky bucket? It might get you through the situation in the here and now, but it's not helping you or your child in the long term, because it's not addressing the root cause of the problem. This means that, at some point, the plaster won't hold on the bucket and the leak will start again.

An alternative approach to managing negative behaviour

Instead of just responding to the behaviour or the actions that we see, we can start to look at and understand the feelings and thoughts that have led to that behaviour. This can be incredibly difficult to do in the moment when your child is experiencing big emotions because, often during these times, their amygdala is in full control. As you've learnt, until they have calmed down, they won't be able to access their memory or logical thoughts. Instead, I recommend that you start to look at the feelings and thoughts after they (and you!) have calmed down, ideally after some happy breathing.

Assuming you're calm now, let's explore this a little further. Using the template below I'd like you to pick one area that you know is a trigger for worry or anxiety in your child. Perhaps it is meeting a new group of people, or having to take a test at school, or standing up in assembly. Don't worry about which example you choose because you can do this exercise over and over again. Just pick the example that comes to mind first. We're going to work through this example using the Thoughts à Feelings à Behaviour model to explore the root cause and start to evaluate alternative approaches.

We're going to start at the bottom of the model and work backwards. First of all, capture the behaviours that you see when your child faces this situation. If someone was recording them with a video camera, what would they see? Don't be tempted to think about thoughts or feelings yet, just focus on what behaviour you would see in this situation:

....

....

....

....

....

Next, take a look at what feelings you think these actions demonstrate. Write them down in the section below:

....

....

....

....

....

Finally, what are the thoughts that your child is having that led to these feelings? Write them down below:

....

....

....

....

....

Now, I want you to think about how you have dealt with this situation in the past and check the box next to the appropriate category. In particular I would like you to think about what you have focused on in the moment and immediately after the behaviour to try to calm your child down:

☐ Is it behaviours?
☐ Is it feelings?
☐ Is it thoughts?

Interesting, right?

Don't worry if you've focused mostly on behaviours and/or feelings – you're definitely not alone. This is where most parents reflect that they've spent their energy before they understand and start integrating this model into their approach.

To be clear, I'm not suggesting that you shouldn't deal with the behaviour at all, but I am suggesting that you pick your moment to do so and that you *also* deal with your child's feelings and thoughts. Remember, trying to deal with feelings and thoughts while the big emotions are in full flow and the amygdala is in control just doesn't work and can even make things worse.

Create positive affirmations

Let's take a minute to think about what you can do differently in any situation where the amygdala has taken hold. How can you shift your focus so that you're addressing the behaviours, the feelings *and* the thoughts, and so supporting your child in the long term?

Remember that your child's behaviour is really just a way of them communicating their feelings and thoughts. While it might not look pretty in the moment, they don't always understand how to do this without lashing out. Helping them to develop the language to communicate these thoughts and feelings more appropriately and start to shift them is where the power really lies.

When you can shift their thoughts, you'll shift their emotions and their behaviours. Wherever possible, you need to try to do this before your child faces the intensity of the situation which is causing them to react. We'll stick with the swimming lesson example to explore this further. The time to work on shifting your child's thoughts is not in the changing room of the swimming pool when they're already distressed! Instead, you could try this before you leave the house for the lesson so that you're dealing with the thoughts before their worry has really started to escalate and the amygdala has taken control.

You may have heard of positive affirmations, and these are really helpful strategies to shift thoughts from being negative to being more positive. Below are some examples of simple affirmations that you could use as the basis for shifting your child's negative thoughts about swimming lessons.

Your child may be resistant to start with, but they will get the hang of it and benefit from it with practice. It can really help to have a conversation about this with your child (depending on their age, of course) so that they too understand the power and control that their thoughts have over their behaviours. Explaining the science of our thoughts, just like explaining how our brains work, is a really helpful part of this learning process for your child. Once they understand this they are more likely to use the affirmations tool effectively. Again, remember, you need to do this before they have become upset and before the amygdala has taken hold.

In the swimming lesson example, the affirmations could sound something like this:

* 'I am safe in the water because my swimming teacher has been trained to help me to stay safe in the water.'
* 'I am safe in the water because there is a lifeguard on duty at all times.'
* 'Once I have learnt to swim, which I will, I will always be safe in the water.'

But what about those situations that you can't plan for? Perhaps your child's amygdala takes control when they see a spider or a fly; in these situations they can start to use this same technique by telling themselves calming thoughts such as, 'It can't hurt me' or 'It is totally harmless.'

The truth is that until we can start to help our children manage their thoughts and feelings, we will always just be dealing with their behaviour and, as we've learnt, this is a very short-term solution. Unless we start shifting their thoughts we'll be sticking that old plaster on the leaky bucket for a long time yet!

This focus on the power of our thoughts is why positive thinking as a body of work and an approach has gained so much traction. Positive thoughts really do lead to positive outcomes. Marcus Aurelius summed this up perfectly when he said: 'The happiness of your life depends on the quality of your thoughts.' Good thoughts lead to good feelings and good feelings lead to good behaviours.

Let's note down some situations where you can start to use positive affirmations to help your child:

....

....

....

....

....

The situations in which my child's negative thoughts lead to negative behaviours are:

....

....

Next time this happens, we will try the positive affirmations just before these situations, such as:

....

....

....

....

....

Example affirmations may include (insert which affirmations you could use):

....

....

....

....

....

Here is a really simple formula that you can use for getting started in coming up with affirmations:

When [insert the thing your child worries about] happens, I will be absolutely [insert positive state of mind] because [insert a positive statement about their character] and [insert a positive statement about why the situation isn't really dangerous].

For instance, if your child worries about meeting new groups of people you could say:

When I go to Brownies for the first time, I will be absolutely fine because I have been brave in new situations before and the adults are there to ensure I have a great time and help me make friends.

You've now added two new tools to your parenting tool-kit: learning how to spot when the amygdala is in control and calm it down with happy breathing, and learning how to shift negative thoughts and so impact negative behaviour.

In the next chapter we're going to look at how you can build your child's self-esteem, and you'll be able to see how the techniques you've learnt here will support you in that as well.

Time to recap

* Whether a danger is real or not, your child's amygdala will respond with fight, flight or freeze. When the danger they see is just perceived, happy breathing techniques can help them to move through these moments differently in the future.

* It's so important to be intentional about how you respond to your child when their amygdala is activated. Ensuring you're mindful of the strategies that do and don't work in the moment can transform how your child will react.

* Responding only to your child's behaviour and not considering the thoughts and feelings that have created this behaviour is a short-term solution. To really help your child to shift thoughts that are causing unwanted behaviour, you have to do the work at the thought and feeling level as well. Just having a conversation around

this and using tools like positive affirmations can be really powerful here.

Your digital resources

In the digital resources for this chapter there's a downloadable happy breathing file which you can play whenever you like. I've picked one of the most popular sessions for children called finger breathing, which is the same activity we went through on pages 32–33.

This is a very sensory activity and one that, after a few goes of listening to the audio, your child (and you) can access. Lots of the children in our programme use this technique in the classroom, for example by placing their hands under the desk, and no one even knows they're doing it!

I'm also giving you poster printouts of Team HAP when they are working well together and when they're not. These will be really useful tools when explaining this to your child or your partner!

See page 235 for details on how to access the digital resources.

My Key Learnings

I want you to use this space to draw, capture and solidify your key reflections from this chapter. What are your 'Aha!' moments and what are you going to do with the learning?

....

....

....

....

....

....

....

....

....

....

....

....

....

....

....

....

CHAPTER 2

Celebrate: Understanding Character

'Watch your thoughts, for they become your words,
Watch your words, for they become your actions,
Watch your actions, for they become your habits,
Watch your habits, for they become your character,
Watch your character, for it becomes your destiny.'

Lao Tzu

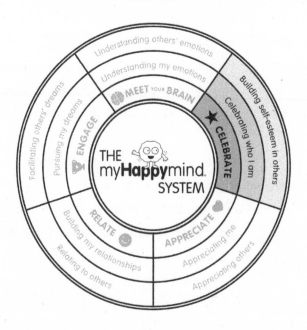

I'm so excited for you to read this chapter! The research into character is one of the most powerful tools that I'll be introducing you to in this book. It's had an incredible impact on the hundreds of thousands of children I work with, and I know it'll impact you and your child too.

Let me start by explaining what 'character' actually means. You're no doubt familiar with the word and will have seen it used in many different ways. Maybe you've described someone as a 'character' meaning they have a big personality. Or perhaps you're just familiar with the word in the context of a film or a TV show.

Well, the way we're going to be thinking and talking about character isn't too far removed from either of these things. When I say character, I am describing someone's character strengths, or the things about them that make them special or unique.

We'll go into some further detail on what character strengths are a little later, but, for now, think of them as things like humour, curiosity and kindness. They are the things that describe who we are as people at our core. They describe the best parts of our personality and the things that come most naturally to us.

Now that we've got a working definition of character, let's explore why it's so important and how it impacts our well-being and happiness.

Self-esteem and Well-being

Self-esteem is defined as: 'a collection of beliefs or feelings that we have about ourselves'. In other words, it is how much we like ourselves.

Self-esteem or how we feel about ourselves is one of the areas that we know is central to our mental well-being and happiness. Put simply, how much we like ourselves, or the level of self-esteem we have, is directly linked to our happiness.

High self-esteem = happier people
Low self-esteem = less happy people

So, what is the relationship between character strengths and self-esteem?

The short answer is that the extent to which we understand and use our character strengths is directly correlated to our self-esteem. In other words, when we understand and use our character strengths, we have higher self-esteem; when we don't, it's lower.

It's clear, therefore, that building self-esteem as much as possible is a really helpful tool in building children's happiness.

How do we build self-esteem?

I'm going to start by summarising how most of the parents I work with (before learning what you're about to learn) would answer this question. They'd likely say that the way they're building their child's self-esteem is to praise their achievements or the things they accomplish. They do this by saying 'well done' and rewarding them for good performance or for achieving things. When a child does well in their spelling test, for example, they'd say something like: 'You're so clever, well done. Let's go to the toy shop and get a treat!' Or, if they get picked for a sports team, they might say: 'You are so sporty, that is brilliant! Shall we go for a milkshake to celebrate?'

The thing that both of these examples of praise have in common is that the focus is on the child's competence or ability. They both focus on what the child is able to *do*.

Now you might be thinking, yes, this is how I build my child's self-esteem too. And if you are, you wouldn't be alone. Most parents think that praising their children for their achievements and then rewarding them is the right way to build self-esteem. When we take a moment to consider what society values and rewards, it's hardly surprising that, as parents, we often focus on these areas of competence or ability. Let's take schools, for example, or education in general: we are rewarded if we achieve high grades or when we learn to *do* something. If we are considered to be *doing* well, we get a good result or grade, and this leads to praise. So, as children, we are recognised and praised for competence-based activity like being good at maths or sport, etc. It's no wonder then that children start to believe that to win praise they need to be 'competent' at things.

Did you experience this as a child? What was your experience growing up of receiving praise at school and at home? Was it based on what you did or were able to do?

It is useful and important to reflect on this as, often, and usually unknowingly, we can carry whatever our experience was into how we parent our own children.

If we consider the workplace it's a similar story. We're set objectives which are typically to do with what we need to 'do' or achieve which, in turn, relies on our competence or ability. If we do well, we're rewarded with a pay rise, a bonus or a positive performance review. Again, we're being conditioned to believe that our performance and competence are the most important things when it comes to being praised or rewarded.

We can see why, as parents, we may be focused mostly on rewarding and praising children's competence or abil-ity as it's what many of us were used to growing up. But here's what the science tells us about how this competence-based approach impacts self-esteem: when we only focus on praising a child's achievement from a competence per-spective, as in the examples above, we actually run the risk of damaging their self-esteem. What? I hear you cry! Stay with me here a minute because this is kind of a big deal and often a revelation to parents . . .

The way that we actually build a child's (or anyone's!) self-esteem is not *just* by praising their achievements from a competence perspective i.e. what they are able to do. Instead, it's to ensure that we praise their character strengths as well as their competence. We must focus on character as much and if not more than we do on competence if we want to build our child's self-esteem.

Praising a child for who they are *being*, or their character, is what builds self-esteem. Just praising a child for what they are *doing* can actually have the opposite effect. Let that sink in for a minute . . .

> *Just praising your child's achievements alone will* not *build their self-esteem.*

Character- versus competence-based praise

You can see now that it is important for us to recognise *how* a child does things and not just *what* they do. I am by no means saying that as parents we shouldn't recognise their achievements; I am saying that we must do this *alongside* praising the character strength or how they are being.

In order to ensure that we move towards a character-based model of praise rather than just a competence-based one, we must first develop our understanding of character strengths. But before we do this, I want to be clear about something that can trip parents up: I'm not saying that you should never notice when you child achieves something – of course you should. Instead, it's *how* you praise them and their achievements that is really important. Let's take a look at those examples from earlier and see how some simple shifts can turn these statements from competence-based praise to integrating character-based praise too:

Competence-based praise	Character- and competence-based praise
'You are so clever, well done. Let's go to the toy shop and get a treat!'	'You really persevered and focused to remember those spellings and your hard work and practice paid off, well done. How would you like to celebrate?'
'You are so sporty, that is brilliant! Shall we go for a milkshake to celebrate?'	'Your determination, practice and focus on being a team player means you got picked – that is fabulous! How would you like to celebrate?'

You can see the subtle difference here, right? Instead of focusing on the outcome or the result, you are focused on the character strength that they used to get that result.

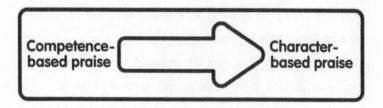

Competence-based praise → Character-based praise

This difference is important because you're reinforcing that they have the character strengths to do these things and so they can do them again. You are not focusing on rewarding what they can do; you are rewarding and praising who they are. This distinction is so critical because of what we believe makes us worthy of praise and love. Let's explore this some more.

To illustrate this point, I'm going to use some extreme scenarios because, while I suspect no child falls on either side of this spectrum, it's helpful to use extremes to really see what we're getting at.

Scenario 1: Competence-based praise

Let's imagine a child who has grown up in a house where their parents focus the majority of their praise around competence. Things like doing well in tests, drawing nice pictures, being good at sport, etc. They only ever give their child praise when they do these things (remember we're dealing in extremes here), so they do not praise their child for their character, for example being kind or caring or curious.

This child will learn through their experience that they are only worth of praise, reward and ultimately love if they accomplish something. This child will have a definition of self which is based solely on their ability or competence. Their self-esteem or how much they like themselves is based on what they are able to do, or their competence. If the child is doing well, for example at school, they will likely get praise and reward at home and so feel good about themselves – this is great right?

But what happens when they're having a tough time with their work or they don't make the sports team? In these scenarios the child may not be getting the praise and acknowledgement at home and, all of a sudden, they start to doubt their self-worth. When they have a bad test (which they're bound to!) or they're asked to do something which they find tricky, they experience this as a knock to their self-esteem. This is because their definition of self is based around their competence. When they perform, they get praise and love; when they don't perform, they don't. Obviously, we want to avoid this at all costs.

Let's take a look at the other side of this spectrum.

Scenario 2: Character-based praise

In this scenario we're going to imagine that the child is mostly praised or rewarded for their character or who they are.

They grow up receiving praise for the *way* in which they do things or for the character traits they are displaying. For instance, 'Well done for using your curiosity to do that piece of research' or 'Look at how determined you were to learn that song for school.'

This child's definition of self becomes one which is based around their character. They believe that they are deserving of love and praise when they display their character strengths or their true self. This in turn leads to them feeling good about who they are and so what follows is high self-esteem.

Therefore, if they have a bad day or don't do so well in a test, they don't have the same response as the child in the first scenario, which was to interpret this as a knock to their self-esteem. Why? Because this child believes that their self-worth is based on their character, not what they achieve.

You can now see how different these definitions of self are, right?

One definition leads to a child who is focused on using their positive character strengths to get praise, while the other leads to a child who is just focused on performance (perhaps at any cost) to get praise. Ultimately, we're all seeking that approval, affirmation and praise, and where we look for it will depend on how we define ourselves.

Now that we've explored the difference between a competence- and a character-based approach to praise, you're probably wondering how you can build this into how you talk to your child. This all begins with understanding more about character strengths.

Exploring Character Strengths

One of the most interesting things about character strengths is that some of them come from our parents or our genetics and some of them come from our experiences.

On the whole debate of 'nature versus nurture', from a character perspective we can safely say, based on the science, that it's a little bit of both. I know this is an interesting one for many parents because often they'll say, 'I just don't understand why my child behaves in that way' or has that character trait.

I often talk to friends or people who I coach, and they'll say: 'I've raised my kids in exactly the same way. Why are they so different?' The answer to this is that our child's character is going to develop partly based on their genetics and partly based on their experiences. Even if you have parented in exactly the same way (which I think we rarely do), the experiences that your children have will be different and so their character will evolve and be different too.

The research

The research into character is thorough and robust. There are a vast number of different models and ways of looking at character and I've studied most of them extensively. They all have different nuances and pros and cons, but the one I've found to be the most robust in terms of its data and methodology is called the 'VIA model'.[1]

This model describes character strengths as:

'the positive parts of your personality that impact how you think, feel and behave. Your character strengths are the qualities that come most naturally to you. When you know your strengths, you can improve your life and thrive. Research reveals that people who use their strengths a lot are 18x more likely to be flourishing than those who do not use their strengths.'

This model is based on the work of Martin Seligman who has, for many decades, extensively researched and studied the science of character. He is a particular hero of mine and I can thoroughly recommend his books for a deeper look into this area.

Seligman is the leader of a movement called 'positive psychology' which asks the fundamental question: 'Rather than focusing on what's wrong with people, why don't we focus on what's right with them?' Positive psychology is a science of the positive aspects of our life, such as our happiness, well-being and flourishing. Seligman and Csikszentmihalyi describe it as 'the scientific study of positive human functioning and flourishing on multiple levels that include the biological, personal, relational, institutional, cultural, and global dimensions of life'.[2] This refreshing approach leads us to put people's strengths at the heart of our thinking about them, rather than looking at where they might need to improve. This becomes particularly powerful in the context of children because, as parents, we can often find ourselves looking at the areas they need to work on. When we focus on our child's character strengths, or what comes to them naturally, we're focusing on what makes them who they are and, as we've already learnt, focusing on character alongside competence is important for our self-esteem and happiness.

It's worth noting here that, as parents, we can fall into the trap of noticing elements of our children's character that are perhaps less positive, for example 'they are bossy' or 'they are just so lazy'. While these might be considered character traits, we must avoid using statements and labelling children like this as it can damage a child's self-esteem. Focusing on the positive elements of their character is what is most important here.

The science behind character is absolutely fascinating. This research has included many neuroimaging studies (where we see what happens in the brain when we use our character strengths) and lots of other research experiments. What these studies consistently show is that when we use our character strengths, we get dopamine released in the brain.

Remember dopamine? It's the feel-good hormone we learnt about in the last chapter (page 37), and it makes us feel happy. So, when we use our character strengths, we feel happy – pretty simple, right? Dopamine also plays a positive role in motivation, reward and pleasure – there's really no downside to it!

We know that using our character strengths makes us feel good (because it releases dopamine) and we also know that when we feel good, we do good. When we feel happier and we're in a state of positive emotion, we do better at everything: work, school, sport, relationships. When we have a positive state of mind, we will perform better in every area of our life. Why wouldn't we want to have more of that in our life?

In order to build your understanding of strengths so that you can integrate this into your parenting toolkit, it's important to learn more about your own strengths. Before we dive into this though, I'd like to set the scene by sharing a little bit more about the research into character strengths.

The VIA model

The study of character strengths started in the early 2000s, when scientists gathered to study character more scientifically. A total of 55 distinguished scientists joined the study over several years. The result was the 'VIA Classification of Character Strengths and Virtues' – a classification of positive traits (character strengths) in human beings. Since then, hundreds of peer-reviewed articles have been published across many cultures about this model.

Once the VIA Classification was complete, a groundbreaking personal strengths test – the VIA Survey – was designed specifically to measure these character strengths in individuals. Since then, over 11 million surveys have been taken around the world and VIA continues to fuel the advancement of character strengths science through research, personalised reports, books and more. This is why I believe this to be the most robust tool when it comes to understanding our character strengths.

This model shows that we are all born with 24 character strengths. Each and every one of us has all 24 strengths no matter where we're from, our religion, our race or our social demographic.

These character strengths are things like kindness, bravery, curiosity, determination and love of learning. They're very much innate strengths or a description of who we are at our core – they are absolutely *not* about competence. This model does not tell you if you are good at maths or science or sport. Again, we're not focused on our ability here at all; we're talking about those characteristics that describe the best parts of your personality.

While we all have all 24 strengths, we'll each have them in different amounts. This means that my most dominant strengths are likely to be different to yours. Remember, this doesn't mean that I don't have all 24 strengths – I just don't use them as much or they're not as strong in me right now.

It's really important to remember that all of these 24 strengths are positive and so, whatever your character strengths profile looks like, you are fabulous!

We are all truly one of a kind: the number of potential character strengths profiles is exponentially greater than the number of people living on our planet.

This is one of the fundamental reasons why I love this tool because, rather than focusing on better or worse, good or bad, or less or more, it just focuses on our strengths, and so it's a really lovely tool to use, both with adults and with children.

Let's Discover Your Strengths!

I believe that in order for you to start identifying and talking to your child about their strengths, it is critical that you understand your own. It is only when you've identified your own strengths that you can really start to embed this approach with your child. There are a number of ways for you to do this but, for now, I am going to walk you through an exercise that will allow you to start to identify your own character strengths.

Celebrate: Understanding Character

I'd like you to consider what you think your strengths are – remember we are talking about character strengths here and not competence. To help you to do this you can use the following questions:

★ How would my partner or friends describe me?
★ What do I get compliments about as it relates to my personality?
★ When faced with a problem, what things help me to get through it?

These prompts should help you to flush out some of your most natural and dominant character strengths. Don't overthink this; just see what comes up for you and jot them down below:

....

....

....

....

....

Next we're going to explore how you use your strengths right now and where you may have opportunities to use them even more. When have you used your top strengths in the last few days?

....

....

....

....

....

Think of a recent big change in your life – it may have been a job change or moving to a new house or a relationship change. How did you use your strengths during this situation?

....

....

....

....

....

Are there any other strengths that would have helped you in this situation? If so, which ones and why?

....

....

....

....

....

Celebrate: Understanding Character

Now that you've explored your top strengths, list your top five below as a reminder:

....

....

....

....

....

OK, how was that? Easy? Tricky? How difficult or not you found this may be an indication of how in tune or not you are with your strengths, but let me say this: *most* people have no idea what their character strengths are because, as we explored right at the start of this chapter, we don't tend to focus on them as a society. We're much more geared towards competence or the things that we are good at doing, but that is all about to change, for you and your family anyway.

Charles Caleb Colton said, 'The true measure of your character is what you do when nobody's watching.' This is a great quote to explain character really simply. It says that our character is who we are when we are in a totally relaxed state. We're not thinking about how we should be behaving or how we might be perceived, we're just being who we are.

This is also a useful way to think about strengths in your child. How do they behave in play or when they are totally relaxed? This can be a great question to think about when identifying their character strengths.

Go even deeper by taking the VIA strengths survey

If you would like to really get under the skin of your strengths I would encourage you to take the VIA strengths survey, which you can find on their website: https://viacharacter.org. Below are some tip tips if you decide to take this or any other survey:

- Don't try to second-guess the answers. (I'm not saying *you* will . . . but some definitely will!) There are no right or wrong answers and so there's no point in trying to game it . . . OK?
- Go with your gut – don't spend too long overthinking the answer, just go with what feels right.
- Take the survey when you have 10 minutes where you won't get distracted. It shouldn't take longer than that to complete.
- If you can print out your results even better!

And remember, whatever your results are:

- You have all 24 strengths – even the ones that are lower down the list – so please don't get distracted by what is at the bottom! Instead, focus on your strengths or what's at the top!

- This is a point-in-time assessment – your strengths can change and grow over time.

- You have all 24 strengths – even the ones that are lower down the list – so please don't get distracted by what is at the bottom! Focus on your strengths or what's at the top! (No, this isn't a typo – I wrote it twice because it's so important!)

How to use your character strengths

Are you starting to see how your strengths have such an impact on how you see and respond to the world? Here are my three top tips on how you can use your new knowledge of the character strengths you've uncovered to boost your own happiness and well-being:

1. Figure out how you can use your strengths more. When you are using your top strengths, you'll be in flow or a state of happiness (see page 90). The more we can use our strengths the better, so seek out as many opportunities as you can to use your top strengths in all of the different roles that you play in life. For instance, can you use your strengths more as a parent? Can you use them more in work? What about in social

situations? The more you use your strengths, the more dopamine you'll release and the happier you'll feel (see page 37)!

2. Celebrate your strengths. Take some time to reflect on how you are using your strengths each and every day. Whether you start a journal or just think about it, keeping strengths top of your mind is a good way to increase your use of them. When we celebrate our strengths we are actually reminding ourselves of the power of them. If we use them and then move on without recognising them, we'll get less of a well-being benefit. Celebrating them can be as simple as having a chat with yourself where you say 'Thank goodness I have bravery as a top strength as I was able to challenge my boss today and get the outcome I wanted.'

3. Notice other people's strengths, including those of your friends, work colleagues, partner, family members and especially your child! (More on that in a minute.) The act of noticing strengths in others will help to solidify your understanding even more. Additionally, when we notice someone else's strengths and tell them that we've noticed them, guess what gets released in their brain? Yes, dopamine! When someone else recognises our strengths, it is the ultimate self-esteem-building compliment because they are essentially saying, 'You are awesome', and who doesn't want to hear that?!

Celebrate: Understanding Character

Now that you have this grounding in the science of character and you've reflected on your own strengths, let's talk about how you can integrate all of this into working with your child.

Celebrating Your Child's Strengths

As we start to think about using a strengths-based parenting approach with your child, we'll begin by taking some time to think about what their strengths are (much like we've just done with you).

To support you in this, I've shared my simplified version of character strengths that we use in our programme. By grouping the character strengths into smaller categories like this, they're easier to use with children. (I've given you a copy of this model in your digital resources – see page 235.) While these five strengths will provide a great starting point, don't feel restricted by them. If there is a strength you see in your child that isn't captured here, please do use this as well. Just remember to apply the following test with yourself: 'Is this definitely a character strength – i.e. how they are being – or is it a competence – i.e. what they are able to do?' This is an adjustment that can take a while, but if you keep asking yourself this question, you'll definitely get there.

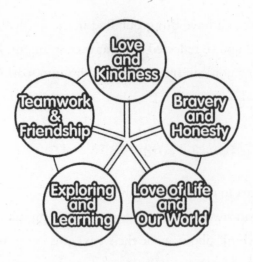

The key to integrating this character work into your parenting is actually wonderfully simple and follows three key steps:

1. Notice them.
2. Comment on them.
3. Celebrate them.

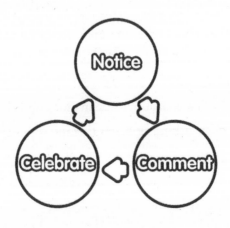

Wait, it's that easy? Yes! Let's take a look at each of these in turn:

Notice them

This might sound really obvious, but it's an incredibly important step. It may take you some time to actually notice and figure out what your child's strengths are and that's OK.

The easiest way to do this is just to observe them and watch how they approach life: what they do, what they say and how they problem-solve. You'll soon start to see some patterns emerge which will then help you to identify their strengths. Don't rush this stage, it isn't a race.

Comment on them

This stage is all about making sure that you don't just notice your child's strengths but that you actually comment on them too. For instance, if you see your child being particularly kind, say to them, 'I'm so pleased to see how kind you're being. That's a real strength of yours. See how it helped your friend?'

You'll notice in this example that we've commented on the strength *and* the outcome this strength has produced. This is really important as you'll then start to solidify your child's understanding of how their strengths help them.

I know that this might feel a little unnatural or almost staged, but you'll soon get into the habit of it the more you do it. Don't feel that you have to notice every single strength every time your child does anything – even noticing three or four things a day consistently will start to shift your child's definition of self.

Celebrate their strengths

This is where it all comes to life. Noticing and commenting on your child's strengths is of course incredibly important, but what really helps to build their self-esteem is when you take time to celebrate their strengths.

For some parents this does involve breaking some habits, like only rewarding and praising your child based on their achievements or competence. This will take some time, but it's incredibly important that you genuinely celebrate the *how* your child achieves and not just the *what* they achieve. For example, if you notice that your child has really persevered in order to achieve a piece of homework, focus on celebrating that perseverance strength rather than the homework outcome. It is also critical to notice your child's character strengths even when they don't achieve, because we don't want them to think that they only receive praise when they achieve.

This subtle shift is absolutely key to helping your child to really believe that their self-worth is based on their character and not just their competence.

You may find it helpful to take a few minutes now to reflect on what some of your child's strengths might be.

Celebrate: Understanding Character

This will help you to accelerate the process of getting into the habit of Notice → Comment → Celebrate.

My child's character strengths are:

....

....

....

....

....

When do I see them using these strengths?

....

....

....

....

....

Now you know what your child's strengths are, it's time to look at how you can bring them to life through everyday situations. Remember there are three key ways to start bringing strengths to the forefront of your parenting: noticing, commenting and celebrating. Let's look at an example here to bring this to life.

Imagine your child is working really hard to revise for a test and there's a lot riding on it (in their eyes at least). When you *notice* them focusing on getting ready for the test you could *comment* on the fact that they are showing the strengths of commitment, focus and diligence and then *celebrate* the fact that these strengths will not only help them in this situation but in others too. You're de-emphasising the fact that they're revising for a competence-based test and emphasising the fact that they are using their strengths which they can apply to other areas too.

You can also use strengths to help your child when they're feeling less sure about a certain situation. By reminding them that they have the strengths to get through the situation, you'll give them confidence and help to remind them of their strengths. I work with a lot of children in their transition from primary school to secondary school, which is often a tricky time. The biggest worry that I hear is 'Will I make any friends?' Here's how I use a strengths-based approach to deal with this common concern.

Firstly, I ask the child what their top strengths are. Let's say they respond with humour, bravery and curiosity. Next, I guide them through a process to look at how they can use these strengths to make friends. They may say, 'I guess I could make a joke in the playground which will make people laugh' and I'll say, 'Yes, perfect – you can use your humour strength to break the ice and start a connection.' Or they might say, 'I could just go over to someone who looks nice and say "Hi"'. Again I would then show them that this is their bravery strength coming into play.

How to develop your strengths

Inevitably when you were reflecting on your own strengths and those of your child you will have considered some strengths that you wish you or they had more of. It is human nature to have this response. While I wholeheartedly encourage you to spend 90 per cent of your focus on thinking about how you can use and celebrate your top strengths more, you can also seek to develop some of the strengths that are less dominant for you and your child.

My advice though is that you just pick one strength at a time to work on, otherwise you'll fall into overwhelm and spend too much time focusing on growth and not enough on celebrating, and getting that balance right is really important.

As you start to consider which strengths you wish you or your child had more of, it's really helpful to think of your strengths like muscles – the more you use them, the more they grow. As we discussed, some strengths come from genetics and some from our experiences, so those strengths that come from our experiences have developed because we've had to practise using them.

This muscle analogy can be a really helpful one when talking to your child. If there is a particular strength that you think they'd benefit from working on, for example perseverance, it's absolutely critical they understand that they can grow this strength with practice. For example, let's say that they have just learnt to ride their scooter. You could explain to them that they used perseverance to achieve this because they had to keep practising over and over again. You could then tell them that in order to build their perseverance strength even more, they can learn other new things that require them to practise or persevere, like riding a bike. Helping children to see that they do already have the strength and that they just need to practise using it to make it stronger is a really powerful strategy to use.

Remember to just focus on growing one strength at a time so this doesn't take over and becoming overwhelming! And, of course, any focus on growing strength should be absolutely complemented by lots of celebrating the top strengths that your child already has!

I hope you can see that by helping your child to think through how they problem-solve and then pulling out their strengths for them, you can bring this strengths-based parenting approach to life.

I'd like to share a story here about one of the parents in our 'Families' programme whose little girl used to be so shy that she wouldn't join any after-school clubs, despite really wanting to. Every time she was in a new situation she would clam up and not be able to speak or join in. Her parents had tried lots of different strategies to support her – from telling her she had to go (tough love, or so they thought) to staying with her and encouraging her – but nothing seemed to work.

When they learnt about this notion of growing strengths they realised that they needed to support her in growing her bravery strength so that she could learn to cope with these situations on her own.

To do this, they first laid some groundwork with her to show her that she has this strength already. They thought of and discussed lots of examples of when she had used her bravery strength before, for example, when performing in the school play or on her first day of school. She started to realise that she does have the bravery strength but perhaps she just doesn't use it as much as she could. Next they started to think about some goals she could set to use her bravery strength even more. She set herself the big goal of joining an after-school club the following term and then set a whole load of mini goals along the way. These all included using her bravery strength. For example, one was to talk to a friend who was already in the club about her favourite parts of it. Another was to be brave enough to ask the teacher who ran the club what activities they would be doing. By setting up these mini goals, all of which required her to use her bravery strength, she was able to build this muscle and see just how much bravery she really has. And guess how it ended? That's right! By the time it got to signing up for the club she did it and had the best time.

By coaching her through this, we gave her the evidence that she already has the bravery strength, but just needed to use it a little more for it to grow. This approach of showing the child they've used the strength before and then helping them to set mini goals to use it even more can be applied to growing any of the strengths and it is really powerful.

Being in 'flow'

Have you ever heard of being in 'flow' state? Some people describe it as being in 'the zone'. You've probably experienced being in a flow state at some point in your life. It's characterised by being totally absorbed in a task or activity and your focus just can't be shaken. Time feels like it's slowed down and you're effortlessly moving through the task or the situation. For you, this might be reading a book or maybe going for a run. And for your child you may notice them getting into this flow state when they're playing with their Lego or perhaps when they're colouring. This will be different for all children but I am sure you'll know some of the times when this happens for yours. Positive psychologist Mihaly Csikszentmihalyi said in a 2004 TED Talk: 'There's this focus that, once it becomes intense, leads to a sense of ecstasy, a sense of clarity: you know exactly what you want to do from one moment to the other.'

Celebrate: Understanding Character

You won't be surprised to hear that being in this flow state is really good for us, and we're likely to be really happy and motivated when we're in it. The more we use our character strengths, the more likely we are to get into this flow state. If you think about the times when you have been in a flow state or in the zone, this may give you some clues as to what your character strengths are.

Why not note them down below? What are the situations where you feel totally in the zone and the activity or task you're doing is just effortless?

....

....

....

What about your child; when do you see them in their flow state?

....

....

....

Have a think about how you can create more space for yourself and your child to be in this flow state more of the time. When you and they are in this state, you'll be able to reap those happiness rewards even more.

The Benefits of Strengths-based Parenting

'Flourishing is like supercharging your well-being and happiness.'

Dr Ryan Niemiec

Ultimately, in order to help children to be happy we want to help them flourish. The good news is that there is more and more research that confirms that shifting to a character-led approach to parenting has a major role in flourishing our children's happiness.

Martin Seligman says: 'These twenty-four strengths underpin all five elements (of happiness), not just engagement: deploying your highest strengths leads to more positive emotions, to more meaning, to more accomplishment, and to better relationships.'[3]

Dr Lea Waters, a leader in the field of positive psychology, says: 'The key to becoming a strength-based parent is to form the habit of swapping the question "What needs to be fixed?" with "What strengths are needed to handle this situation?" In other words, flipping the Strength Switch.'[4]

The benefits of a strengths-based approach to parenting are far-ranging, but the following are three of the most powerful ones:

1. It helps children reach their full potential

When we focus on our strengths (rather than our weaknesses or areas of potential improvement) we get better at things. Olympic athletes didn't get those medals because they focused on their weaknesses; they got them because they focused on and leveraged their strengths. Therefore, our children's route to achieving their full potential is not through focusing on those areas that they find challenging, but instead it is through focusing on their strengths. This builds their self-esteem and helps them to excel in the areas that they are most passionate about.

2. It builds children's well-being

When we encourage children to use their strengths to problem-solve and navigate the world around them, their life satisfaction, self-confidence and overall positive emotions are higher. Further, children with parents who take a strength-based approach show less stress, fewer issues with managing friendship problems and they do better academically. This strengths-based approach to parenting has also been shown to prevent depression, bullying and underachievement in children.

3. It fosters a good relationship between the child and the parent

By focusing on your child's strengths you are able to find more opportunities to celebrate and connect with your child. This teaches you as their parent to see the best in your child and ultimately this in turn builds trust and better relationships between you.

This all sounds pretty good, right? If you weren't already convinced about the merits of a strengths-based parenting approach, I'm pretty sure you will be now!

The next chapter is focused all around the incredible power of gratitude and how you can implement this into your everyday rituals to not only boost your child's happiness but to also build their resilience.

Time to recap

* Our children's strengths come partly from genetics and partly from experiences. This shows that strengths are things that we can grow. We all have all of the strengths (no matter what our social, economic, religious or nationality status may be); we just have them in different amounts.

* When you understand your own strengths you are more able to support your child in understanding theirs. If you skipped this step (no judgement here!), I'd really recommend that you go back and complete the exercise now (page 85).

* The approach of 'noticing, commenting and celebrating' is a powerfully simple way to get started in using

strengths-based parenting, as well as using problem-solving as a way to tease out your child's strengths.

★ You can use your understanding of your child's strengths as the basis for shifting to a more balanced approach to praise. By focusing on both competence- and character-based praise, you're able to ensure that your child feels good about who they are at their core and that they do not become obsessed and defined by their competence or their ability.

★ If children have high self-esteem and feel good about who they are, they'll be happier and more resilient in the face of challenge and ride through this journey we call life so much more smoothly.

Your digital resources

One of the most powerful things to help make character become part of your everyday conversations with your child is just to keep it at the top of your mind! A gentle visual 'nudge' to remind you to focus on character and competence is super powerful. That's why I'm giving you a gorgeous printable poster to remind you about the importance of character. Print this out and put it on your fridge or in your office, or wherever you'll see it the most. Visual cues are super helpful, particularly when we're shifting our everyday language, so I really hope this helps you.

I'm also giving you a poster of the simplified strengths we use in our programme to help you to use this with your child.

See page 235 for details on how to access the digital resources.

My Key Learnings

I want you to use this space to draw, capture and solidify your key reflections from this chapter. What are your 'Aha!' moments and what are you going to do with the learning?

....
....
....
....
....
....
....
....
....
....
....
....
....
....
....

CHAPTER 3

Appreciate: Gratitude

*'Feeling gratitude and not expressing it is like
wrapping a present and not giving it.'*
William Arthur Ward

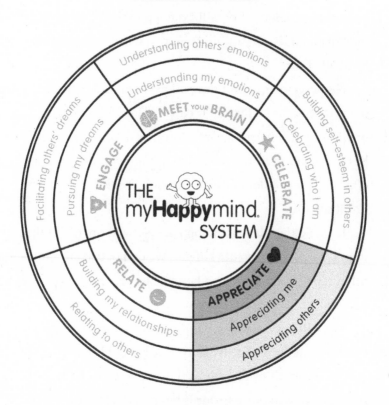

This next part of the myHappymind system is wonderfully simple but incredibly powerful. It focuses on the huge shifts that developing a true gratitude habit can have on children's well-being and happiness, as well as how gratitude helps to build resilience.

One of the things I have often observed children and adults saying is: 'I'll be happy when [insert any number of reasons why]'. People often attach some kind of physical goal or destination to being happy, such as, 'I'll be happy when I get that promotion' or 'I'll be happy when I have all of the Pokémon teddies' or 'I'll be happy when I get a remote-controlled car.'

However, what we know about happiness is that it is not a destination. Happiness can't be found by aspiring to a thing or a particular circumstance. Instead, happiness has to be found in the present-day moment and the most effective way of doing this is through regularly practising gratitude.

It is said that 'It is not happy people who are grateful; it is grateful people who are happy.' We do not become grateful as a by-product of being happy. We become happy as a by-product of practising gratitude.

We will never achieve happiness if we are always striving for something that we don't yet have. However, if we can focus on all of the things that we have to be grateful for now, we will move towards happiness. Happiness is not found in the future, it is found in the here and now and it all begins with gratitude.

Appreciate: Gratitude

For those of you who share my love of stationery you may have noticed the rise of gratitude journals or notebooks with gratitude quotes on the front of them in your favourite stationery store. Am I right? Or, if stationery isn't your thing but you're on social media, it's likely that you've seen lots of gratitude quotes popping up on Instagram and Facebook.

Over the last decade or so there have been a number of landmark studies that have shown the true power of gratitude. This deepened understanding, along with advances in technology like brain scanners, has meant that scientists have been able to evidence how gratitude positively impacts our well-being and happiness by directly looking at the effect it has on our brains.

Let's start by understanding a bit more about these research studies, what they tell us and why they matter. The dictionary definition of gratitude is: 'The quality of being thankful and a tendency to show appreciation for what one has.'

The first research study I want to share is by psychologists Emmons and McCullough.[1] They sought to explore how the simple act of just writing the things down that we're grateful for affects our happiness. Essentially, they wanted to answer the question – can journaling about our gratitude really help us be happier?

In order to explore and answer this question they conducted a research study involving three groups of people.

Each group was invited to capture something different about their week. The first group was asked to capture five things they were grateful for; the second was asked to capture what had irritated them; and the third noted events that had impacted them that week.

Here's what the results showed. The people who had taken time to be grateful each day were much happier and more positive than those who had focused on hassles or events. In addition, there were some other unexpected outcomes between the group that had focused on gratitude and the other two groups. As well as having higher levels of happiness and positivity, this group was also more likely to:

* Exercise for more time each week than the other two groups. Being grateful, which leads to greater mental well-being, also makes us more motivated to look after ourselves physically.

* Have a positive outlook about the future, even in the short term, for example, about their upcoming week. By being grateful for all that they have now, they were able to have more optimistic thoughts about their future possibilities too.

* Experience less physical pain or illness. This study showed that those who were focused on all they had to be grateful for felt less physical pain or illness than

those who were focused on the negative elements in their lives.

What we can see from this is that gratitude has incredible benefits for our happiness and overall well-being. Given this, I'd now like to turn your thoughts to how much of a gratitude mindset you bring to your everyday life.

How often are you thinking about and expressing gratitude? Do you look back on your week and think about all you have to be grateful for, or are you someone who tends to focus more on the hassles or what didn't go so well?

I'm posing these questions because they are so critical as we think about happiness. Our thoughts matter, and where we focus them clearly impacts our happiness. In turn, the extent to which we as parents role model thinking about all that we have to be grateful for versus all that is wrong in the world, will have a huge impact on how our children's thinking habits will develop. It is often said that, 'If you only realised how powerful your thoughts are, you'd never think a negative one again.'

Another study that I think is worthy of note is by Martin Seligman (who we met in the last chapter for his work around character strengths).[2] Seligman wanted to explore how sharing gratitude with someone you're in a relationship with impacts our happiness and that of the other person.

He asked people to write a letter of gratitude to someone who had helped them or who had been especially kind but had never properly been thanked. Again, a pretty simple act, right? Not only did this act of gratitude hugely increase their happiness in the moment, the positive effect lasted for weeks after. This study also showed that the person in receipt of the gratitude letter had immediate and long-lasting positive well-being effects from this interaction too.

Again, something really small that requires very little effort can produce these huge well-being benefits. But why? When I first started researching gratitude, I was really surprised to learn that the amount of dopamine (the feel-good hormone) that gets released in the brain when we give gratitude is very similar to the amount that gets released in the brain when we receive it. So, it turns out that giving and receiving gratitude is really the ultimate win–win, it's great for the giver and the receiver!

This is why the opening quote by William Arthur Ward is so poignant; while feeling gratitude is great (just like receiving a present), we only get the full benefit from it when we share it with the person towards whom we feel it (giving the present). Yet, in our society and in our relationships, we so often fail to actually express our gratitude to others, even when we feel it. For instance, when our child helps us in the house or shares nicely with their friends we might notice it but we don't always express our gratitude for these things. Yet, there are such positive benefits for us and our children when we do.

If we can understand why this is the case, we can start to shift this, express more gratitude and therefore make a lasting impact on our own and our child's well-being.

There are all sorts of reasons why gratitude is less prominent than it could be in our society, but we'll just explore three of the key ones here. Firstly, let's look at the way in which our society or way of life may be impacting our gratitude practice versus how we may have lived just 10 or 20 years ago. Our increasingly fast-paced, instant-access lifestyle means that we can access most things that we want on demand.

It used to be the case that we had to wait a week for the next episode of our favourite TV programme to come out, but now we can simply binge-watch it on Netflix. Or, if we wanted a particular pair of shoes, we'd need to actually go to a shop to buy them, but now we can have them delivered to our door the same day. While it can't be denied that technology has enriched our lives, it's also changed the nature of how we live – we can get pretty much anything on demand, at any time. However, the process of anticipating something and having to wait for it makes us desire it more and so we feel more gratitude when we receive it.

Secondly, we'll look at what psychologists and researchers call the 'curse of knowledge'. This isn't about our ability to feel or experience gratitude, but instead it looks at the fact that when we do feel it, we don't always express it. The 'curse of knowledge' describes a situation where we assume that because we feel gratitude towards someone, they must know that. We know it, so it must be obvious to them too. There is no reason to express the gratitude to them and so we don't. But nothing is ever obvious to others because they can't read our minds! So, we end up not sharing our gratitude and miss the opportunity for greater human connection, and all of the happiness benefits that sharing this gratitude would bring.

Finally, we often feel uncomfortable or 'awkward' when we have to express certain emotions because we aren't exactly sure how to do it or we don't know how the other person will respond. This can lead us to think that if we don't how know to express our feelings of gratitude, then there is no way that the person will understand us if we do share them. In turn, we can end up not saying anything because we fear that we'll make a fool of ourselves. But in this overthinking process we lose the most valuable point of the whole exercise, which is that people don't really care about what we say, they care about the intent behind why we say it – they'd feel the sentiment of your gratitude however confused your actual words might be, and that is what matters. Sometimes we can get so hung up on saying the right thing that we end up saying nothing at all.

Appreciate: Gratitude

Carl W.Buehner put it beautifully when she said, 'people will forget what you said, people will forget what you did, but people will never forget how you made them feel'.

How often do you express gratitude?

Now that we understand more about why people don't use gratitude as much as they could, despite the overwhelming evidence of its benefits, let's look at where you are on this topic. As always, remember that these exercises are for you and no one else, and so it's important to be honest – this is an opportunity to learn and grow, so let's take full advantage of that.

Use the space below to write down your reflections on how much of a role gratitude plays in your life today. Do any of the reasons that we've just explored as to why we don't always express gratitude resonate for you?

....

....

....

....

....

As we move into trying to build even more gratitude into your life, let's capture three things that you feel grateful for right now. Don't overthink this – just write down whatever comes to mind:

....

....

....

What Are You Grateful For?

When I talk to people about gratitude and ask them what they're grateful for they will often mention material possessions first. They might say, 'I'm grateful for my house' or 'I'm grateful for my car' or perhaps if I asked a child they might say 'I'm grateful for my phone or my PS4.' There is nothing wrong with being grateful for things, but what we know is that our happiness doesn't come from having more stuff, so it doesn't make sense for us to focus our gratitude there.

In a moment we'll delve into this a little more so that you can see where we can focus our gratitude so that is does support our happiness. Before we do that, I'd like to quickly share a research study with you that illustrates the impact of having more stuff as it relates to our happiness.

Appreciate: Gratitude

In 2003, researchers and psychologists Van Boven and Gilovich looked into the impact that buying experiences versus buying 'stuff' or material possessions has on our happiness.[3] I want to share their results with you because they shatter the promises advertisers and brands make to us about how 'getting more' stuff will make us feel.

What these researchers found is that we predict that buying stuff will make us happier than spending the same amount of money on an experience. However, the truth is that buying experiences actually makes us happier than buying things. Not only this, but experiences give us a greater well-being effect before, during and after the event, whereas our spike in happiness when we buy something is really just at the moment of purchase. With experiences, we get a happiness benefit while planning, anticipating and then remembering the experience too.

In 2014, psychologist Amit Kumar and his colleagues looked further into anticipating experiences versus anticipating buying stuff and found something quite remarkable.[4] When anticipating buying 'stuff', the emotion we feel is more around an impatience to get it, whereas when we anticipate an experience, the feelings are more around genuine excitement. Even thinking about these experiential events make us happier than thinking about buying things.

This research is incredibly powerful, particularly in the context of our materialistic society as I often hear people yearning for more stuff – that next car, the latest PS4 game, whatever it might be. While there is of course nothing wrong with liking nice things, we should be mindful that it is not getting more things that impacts our happiness. It is having experiences that engender social connections and relationships, which we'll explore further in the next chapter.

Ensuring that children do not become totally obsessed with 'stuff' or material things is one of the first and most powerful things that we can start to focus on with them as it relates to gratitude and their happiness. Are they overly emphasising their material possessions when it comes to the things they express gratitude for? If so, starting to look at drawing their attention to other things in their lives that they can be grateful for will be transformational for them and for you.

Based on this research and what we know about what makes us tick as humans, we very intentionally look at gratitude through some specific categories in the myHappymind system. We emphasise the following three areas and encourage children to focus their attention around these when they're thinking about what they're grateful for – you'll notice that 'stuff' isn't one of them!

1. Gratitude for experiences.
2. Gratitude for others.
3. Gratitude for ourselves.

Appreciate: Gratitude

Often children mirror us when it comes to where they express their gratitude. So, as you read through the next three sections, try to keep in mind the extent to which you and your child focus your thoughts around these categories right now. Being mindful of this will help you to formulate a plan around where you can focus as a family moving forward.

Experiences

As we've learnt, the research shows that we get more happiness from the experiences that we have than from the things that we buy. It follows, then, that when we take time to think about the experiences that we have had we'll feel really good about them. Taking time to notice with your child that you had the experience of going for a picnic because the weather was nice or making a point of talking about the fact that they got to have an unplanned play date because they bumped into their friends at the park are examples of ways in which we can encourage children to feel grateful for the experiences they have had.

We also know from the science that learning to savour our experiences in the moment is a huge factor in how much positive emotion we can extract from them. Savouring is the act of stepping outside of an experience to review and appreciate it.

When we have a positive experience, we can either just live it and move on or we can truly savour it. Savouring an experience means that we consciously think about the reasons why we're enjoying the experience as we're having it. Doing this is shown to intensify and lengthen the positive emotions that come from it.[5]

Savouring may include sharing the experience with another person and thinking about how fortunate you have been to have this experience. In the example of having seen friends at the park your child might say something like: 'I'm so lucky to have seen them in the park because it's so much more fun when we are all together . . .' Or you may choose to keep a souvenir or photo of the experience that you can look back on and share with others. Essentially it is all about trying to stay in the present moment throughout the entire experience and notice every little part of it.

Encouraging your child to savour the experiences they have by talking to them about them will further amplify their ability to feel grateful for the experiences that they have.

Others

When we focus our gratitude around the relationships that we have with other people, we remind ourselves of the positive social connections that we have. Social connection is one of the most fundamental components of our happiness (as we'll explore in the next chapter). By encouraging children to notice those people for whom they're grateful we are helping them to create positive emotions for themselves. For example, if your child has a sleepover at their grandparents' house, you can encourage them to be grateful that their grandparents put so much effort into making it special for them. Then, you can help them to amplify their positive emotions even more by encouraging them to share this gratitude with their grandparents. This not only helps your child to feel more positive emotions but, as we've learnt, it has well-being effects for the receiver of the gratitude too!

Ourselves

This is an interesting area because most of us don't take the time to be grateful for ourselves. We aren't necessarily in the habit of stopping and reflecting on all that we've achieved and, critically, how we've achieved it. Instead we can be in the habit of noticing those things that we're yet to achieve or that are still on our to-do list – this isn't helping anyone, least of all you.

The way in which I encourage parents to think about this with their children is to look at it through the lens of character strengths. Asking questions such as: 'What character strengths have you used today?' or 'How have they helped you?' is a really simple way to focus the mind here.

For instance, if you know that your child used their bravery strength to ask a question at school, you could encourage them to be grateful for having this strength. Or perhaps they tell a joke at the dinner table and you all laugh – you could remind them that they should be grateful for their humour strength because they always make others smile. When we help children to look at themselves through the lens of character, this category of gratitude for yourself becomes much easier to access.

This is a great example of how we can pull different elements of the myHappymind system together and derive even more benefit from each of them. By combining your knowledge of your child's character strengths with taking time to be grateful for yourself, you can really impact their happiness and well-being.

Now that you have a framework for looking at your child's character strengths (see page 85), let's spend a little time practising this last category of gratitude for ourselves through the lens of your child.

Use the space below to capture your child's top three character strengths:

....

....

....

Next I'd like you to think about how they've used each of these character strengths over the last week and reflect on how they helped them or, in other words, why they should be grateful for them.

Appreciate: Gratitude

This will help you to see why your child should be grateful for the character strengths that they have. Don't skip past this exercise, even if you're tempted to! Taking the time to think about and write these things down helps you to learn and start integrating this into your child's everyday life.

....

....

....

....

....

Hopefully this exercise has helped you to start thinking about how you can use character strengths as a way to draw out gratitude for ourselves and you can start to help your child establish this as a habit.

Your Gratitude Audit

Now that we've explored these three categories, or types, of gratitude, we're going to complete what I like to call a 'gratitude audit'. The point of this is to uncover the opportunities that you have to integrate more gratitude into your daily life and that of your child. As we do this, we're going to look at you and your child to try to identify any patterns that might emerge. While you know your child better than anybody, of course you don't know their deepest darkest thoughts. That said, what you can do is notice how often you hear them expressing gratitude against the three categories we've explored above. This will start to give you an idea of where they are now and where you'd like to take them.

How often on average do you take time in the week to be grateful?

....

How often on average does your child take time in the week to be grateful?

....

When you think about what you're grateful for, do you ever think about experiences?

....

When you think about what your child expresses gratitude for, do they ever mention experiences?

....

When you think about what you're grateful for, do you ever think about others?

....

When you think about what your child expresses gratitude for, do they ever mention others?

....

When you think about what you're grateful for, do you ever think about yourself?

....

When you think about what your child expresses gratitude for, do they ever mention themselves?

....

Taking a look at your responses above, where do you think you and your child have opportunities to focus more?

....

....

....

....

Creating a Gratitude Habit with Your Child

Wherever you have landed both in terms of assessing your own gratitude habits and those of your child, one thing is for sure — we can all benefit from feeling and expressing more gratitude. Whether you have a lot of space for growth here or just a little, the great thing is that you can move forward and make progress very quickly.

The gratitude audit you've just completed can become the basis of your plan on how you can start taking some daily action to embed a gratitude habit for you and for your child. In terms of how you do this, there are lots of options and there's no right or wrong here – what matters is that you choose something that you remember to do daily and that your child will engage in too. Here are some strategies that you can try to get you going, but of course, you can come up with your own approaches too.

Role modelling

If gratitude is something that happens in your house as part of your normal family conversations, then guess what? Your child sees you role modelling gratitude by expressing it to them and to others in the house and they'll start to do the same. For example, if you thank your child for keeping the playroom tidy and explain that this saves you a job, they'll notice that and are likely to express gratitude when you do something for them. Or if you tell your child that you are so grateful for their kindness strength because they use it to support their siblings, then they'll start to notice character strengths in others. It's as simple as that.

Often the parents I coach will say to me that their children just don't express gratitude and this really frustrates them because they're so lucky to have all that they do and they get to have so many positive experiences.

I get it. This can be really frustrating. However, it's important that you don't get caught in a trap here. If we deal with this frustration by constantly nagging them to say thank you then this can quickly backfire. Your intent here shouldn't be to just hear the words 'thank you'. Instead, we want to encourage your child to really start to feel gratitude. The quickest and most effective way to help them to become more grateful is not to nag at them to say thank you. Instead, it is to simply start expressing gratitude to them each and every day. This way they will start feeling the benefit of receiving gratitude and get those lovely happy hormones flowing and, with some time, they will start to model this back to you.

Gratitude conversations

Gratitude conversations are simply times when you very intentionally encourage your child to reflect on gratitude. My personal favourite is spending some time, usually in the evening, thinking about what each member of the family is grateful for from that day. This is a particularly nice activity for around the dinner table or as part of the bedtime routine.

Here are some questions you can ask to prompt these conversations:

★ What is one thing that you got to do today that you're grateful for?

★ Which one person do you feel grateful to have in your life today?

★ How did you use your strengths today, how did they help you? (And then you can follow up by saying this is something for them to be grateful for.)

When children go to sleep thinking about all that is good in their world, they sleep so much better, so I definitely recommend having these conversations towards the end of the day. Remember that by having a conversation at bedtime or around the dinner table you are facilitating the process of both giving and receiving gratitude which ensures an even greater happiness effect.

Gratitude diaries

For some, writing down their thoughts as they relate to gratitude is their go-to strategy. This can be as simple as asking your child to write down three things that they're grateful for each day. As we saw in Martin Seligman's study (page 103), this simple act of writing down what we're grateful for is incredibly powerful in the short and in the long term. There are lots of fancy gratitude journals that you can buy, but honestly, the power of this practice is just in writing down and reflecting on things that we are grateful for. So don't feel you need to spend any money on this for it to have an impact.

> **Top tips for gratitude success**
>
> - When we're expressing gratitude to children it's so important to explain what we are grateful for and why. For example, if you choose to express gratitude to them because they helped you dry the dishes, also tell them why this mattered to you by explaining that by helping you they've saved you time and that means you can watch that film together now. When a child understands that you feel gratitude and why you feel that gratitude, they're much more likely to repeat the activity again.
>
> - Remember that there is no such thing as right or wrong when it comes to what your child is grateful for. As parents it can be tempting to apply our view of what they 'should' be grateful for, but this rarely gets authentic results. Though they might say thank you for something, it is unlikely they are really feeling the full gratitude if they're simply saying it to appease you. Instead, support your child in feeling gratitude by allowing them to be on the receiving end of it.

■ Like with any habit, this may take time to establish but you have something very powerful on your side and that is dopamine. Since giving and receiving gratitude releases dopamine, once your child is in the habit of it, it becomes self-sustaining. It's a bit like when you get into a good habit around exercise, you rarely want to go back to never leaving the sofa because exercise makes you feel so good. The good news here, of course, is that when you express gratitude to them, you get the benefits too! Dopamine all around!

I'd like to share the story of one of the families I coach here. Establishing a gratitude habit definitely didn't come easily to them, but now they've cracked it, it has enhanced their family life remarkably. This mum and dad felt their son was just so ungrateful. Whenever they bought him something or did something for him, he would fail to express any gratitude. They were constantly nagging him to be more grateful and say thank you. This wasn't working and, in fact, it was just making him more irritable and closed to sharing his gratitude. I encouraged them to look at how often they were expressing gratitude to him by completing a gratitude audit. To their surprise – and, in their words, horror – they realised that they were very rarely expressing gratitude to him because they were so focused on *his* lack of gratitude!

So, they got to work at intentionally communicating their gratitude to him; they'd express gratitude for him doing his homework with no fuss, for hanging his coat up, for bringing his laundry downstairs. In fact, the more they started looking for things to be grateful to him for, the more they found. Can you guess what started to happen? His mood started to brighten, and he started expressing gratitude back – for the little things, like cooking his dinner, and for the big things, like buying him presents.

This is the power of role modelling; sometimes our children need to *see* us using these strategies before they will start. *Telling* them to do something is not always the best way to get gratitude flowing and this was certainly true for this lovely family.

Fostering Resilience

Before we close this chapter, I want to talk about the wonderful effect that having an established habit of gratitude has on resilience. Resilience is defined in the dictionary as 'the capacity to recover quickly from difficulties;

toughness'. In other words, it refers to our ability to cope when we face tough times.

Resilience is a word you are bound to have heard in the context of your child's school motto or ethos. It is universally accepted that children need to be resilient in order to reach their full potential in life. This is truer than ever given the challenging and dynamic world our children are growing up in. Resilience helps them to push through difficulties, to keep going even when it is tough and, ultimately, to become their best self. We all want that for our children, but how do we help them to develop resilience? We'll explore this some more in Chapter 5, but I do want to share how establishing a habit of gratitude can help you to foster resilience in your child.

When we have an established gratitude habit, and we have a bucket that is 'full' when it comes to gratitude, we tend to cope better with challenging situations. This is because if we feel that, in general, we have a lot to be grateful for and then we have a bad day, it doesn't hit us as hard as when we have a bad day and we're already feeling like life is hard. This makes a lot of sense doesn't it?

Take the example of a child going to school with a full bucket of gratitude. They have an overall sense of well-being which is derived from the fact that they feel good about themselves, their relationships and the experiences that they have. For whatever reason, maybe a squabble with a friend or a test that didn't go so well, they don't have the best day. However, because their outlook is generally rosy (due to their gratitude habit) they can cope with this and bounce back relatively quickly because it doesn't seem like the end of the world to them.

Contrast that with the child whose gratitude bucket is not full. They go to school and have a tough day. As they don't have that overarching sense of well-being this just adds to their woes and so the squabble with their friend or the tricky test feels like a bigger deal. Not only does the event itself impact their happiness more, they don't have that same gratitude bank to draw on to help them bounce back.

Both for children and adults, establishing a gratitude practice (whatever form this takes) is incredibly important for our resilience. It gives us perspective, which in turn allows us to bounce back more quickly.

So far, we've been focused on those areas that can help support our happiness and well-being from an inward-looking perspective – those things that we can do for ourselves. Next we're going to explore the importance of relationships with others and how this is such an important factor in our children's happiness and well-being. By taking this outward-looking perspective, we'll be looking at the critical importance of our social connections.

Time to recap

★ Establishing a gratitude habit is an amazing tool to help children build their happiness and well-being. As the research shows, it has an incredible dopamine-inducing power and the more we use it the happier we'll feel. When we express gratitude, we can create the ultimate win–win experience in which both the giver and the receiver of gratitude reap the benefits.

★ Stuff doesn't make us happy, rather experiences do. If we can turn our gratitude to focusing on those experiences we have, alongside thinking about the people we're grateful for and ourselves, we'll get so much more of the happiness benefits that gratitude provides.

★ When it comes to establishing a gratitude habit with your child there are a number of strategies you can use, including role modelling, gratitude conversations and gratitude diaries. What matters, though, is that you find an approach that works for your family and that you create some intentional time to stick with it.

★ A gratitude habit is about more than just feeling good; it also helps us to build our resilience. When we see the world through the lens of gratitude, we are much better able to cope with the tough times. Gratitude is an incredible tool for giving us perspective and ensuring we're focused on all that is good, as well as those challenges that we may face.

Appreciate: Gratitude

Your digital resources

Gratitude is a habit that, once established, will have a long-lasting and positive effect on your child's happiness. In order to help you get started with it I'm giving you some really simple gratitude prompts to help you to reflect on what you and your child have to be grateful for. These simple prompts will help you to explore what you're grateful for and also help you to facilitate your child thinking about this too.

See page 235 for details on how to access the digital resources.

My Key Learnings

I want you to use this space to draw, capture and solidify your key reflections from this chapter. What are your 'Aha!' moments and what are you going to do with the learning?

....

....

....

....

....

....

....

....

....

....

....

....

....

....

....

....

CHAPTER 4

Relate: Building Positive Relationships

'In the final analysis of our lives – when the to-do lists are no more, when the frenzy is finished – the only thing that will have any lasting value is whether we've loved others and whether they've loved us.'

Oprah Winfrey, *What I Know for Sure*

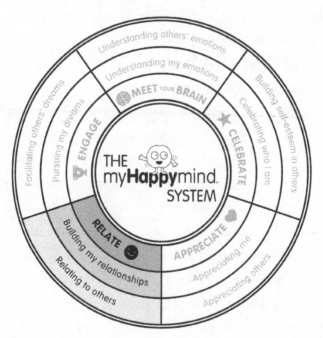

Let's take a few minutes to review all of the incredible strategies that you've already learnt about before we explore the next part of the myHappymind system.

We started our journey by understanding the brain and learning how to notice when it is working well as opposed to when it's stressed. You then took some time to reflect on those amygdala moments which make your child fight, flight or freeze. I really hope that you've been able to notice when these moments happen for your child and that you've started to take a different approach to managing their big emotions. Perhaps you've realised that certain situations – such as bedtime or homework time – really do cause them to go into a fight, flight or freeze response. Tuning in to this and making different choices as to how you support them will become a game changer for you, and for your child. You may have also found yourself noticing when your amygdala activates too!

In Chapter 2 you did some really powerful work to understand what is special and unique about you and your child through the lens of character strengths. And, of course, we took some time to really examine the extent to which you're focused on competence versus character as it relates to how you praise your child. I'm sure by now that you've already started to shift the way that you look at your child in terms of focusing on their character strengths as well as what they're able to do or their competence. Have you started praising their kindness, curiosity or humour? Seeking out and noticing the moments when your child is using their character strengths will be doing wonders for their self-esteem!

Next we delved into gratitude where we really started to focus on slowing down and observing all that we have to be grateful for. We learnt that this isn't just beneficial for us, but for our children and for all those we choose to express gratitude to. As you continue to embed a gratitude habit into your daily lives as a family, you're bound to see how addictive it becomes. The more you and your child give gratitude, the more you'll receive it. This habit will also reap huge well-being and resilience benefits for your child. You'll notice, with time, that they'll have a rosier outlook on life because their gratitude bucket is full, and so they can better cope with knockbacks and challenges.

It's time now to move into 'Relate'. In this chapter we'll really start to look at the role relationships play in our happiness and how you can support your child in developing relationship-building skills.

The Link between Relationships and Our Happiness

There is a direct link between our overall happiness and the quality of our relationships. You've likely had times in your life when the relationships around you have been positive (I sincerely hope this is where you are now).

During these times you may have had healthy relation-ships with your partner, your family, your work colleagues and your child. It is highly likely that you felt happy and positive about your life as a result of these good relation-ships. Does this resonate for you?

When our relationships are healthy, we tend to feel sup-ported and connected to others in our lives and this also helps us to be more resilient. Even if you or your child are having a hard time, for example with your job or in the playground, if you have positive relationships around you, you're much more able to cope with these times than if you don't.

This is because your relationships become a support network which gives you the strength to feel that you can move past difficulties and sustain hope for the future. Let's say you've had a bad day at the office – maybe a presen-tation you had to give didn't go so well. If you come home to a positive relationship with your partner and your kids, and they comfort you and make you smile, then it's likely that your tough day doesn't seem so bad. Or let's say your child comes home upset because they didn't get picked for the football team. You wrap them up in love, fun and make the evening super special and all of a sudden it doesn't seem so bad for your child.

Sadly, most of us have also had times when our rela-tionships have been less positive. Again, this could be with friends, family, partners, etc. During these times you may well have felt less good about life, maybe you felt lonely or unsupported. Let's take a look at that same example of a presentation not going well for you at work. If you don't have positive relationships to lean on after a bad day then you are likely to go home and wallow in your sadness, which will put more emphasis on the things that aren't going so well for you. And so the cycle continues. The chances are that there have been times when your child has come home from school or nursery upset. Often, the cause of this will have been some kind of friendship issue – maybe they were left out of a game at playtime or they found out that they hadn't been invited to a friend's party. Events like this, which essentially are about relationships, can be devastating for a child but sadly they become part of their daily lives from even the youngest of ages.

The truth is that positive relationships give us perspective, allow us to be more resilient and bounce back from the hard times more easily. When it comes to children, positive relationships act as a soothing blanket when things get tough. This isn't rocket science and may not be that surprising to you. However, while it may be deeply intuitive that the quality of our relationships will impact how happy we are, many of us don't seek to build and manage our relationships accordingly.

Despite the fact that we know that ensuring we have positive relationships in our lives is really important, we can all probably point to times in our lives when we've found ourselves in relationships that weren't that positive. Further, we've probably all had times in our lives when we knew this and didn't act upon it. My intent here is to bring your attention back to the importance of relationships. Then, I want to help you to teach your child some foundational skills in how to build positive relationships. Teaching them these skills will help to establish their relationship-building super-powers so that they can learn how to make and sustain positive friendships. This will allow them to develop positive support networks as well as building their self-esteem and confidence. Giving your child these skills is a lifelong gift that will reap dividends for their happiness and well-being.

Before we start looking at the strategies we can use to build positive relationships, I want to spend a bit of time sharing the science of why relationships are so important to our happiness.

The science of relationships

Many positive psychologists have looked into why social connection or positive relationships are so important to our happiness. They've found in study after study that positive relationships are more important than things like material possessions, salaries and the houses we live in, yet we still don't always prioritise relationships as much as we could.

In 2020, psychologist David Myers completed a study that found that people with close social connections are less vulnerable to premature death, are more likely to survive a fatal illness like cancer and are less likely to fall ill on the back of stressful life events.[1] It's clear that there are some very real and positive physical health benefits from maintaining healthy social connections and relationships.

Another study by psychologists Diener and Seligman in 2000 looked at how positive relationships impact our happiness.[2] They looked at two groups of people: a group that considered themselves to be very happy and a group that considered themselves to be unhappy. What they found is that the people who were very happy tended to have more close friends, strong family ties and more romantic ties. They also found that the happiest people spent more time with friends and people who they have good relationships with.

Having discovered this, the researchers were keen to understand whether they could use these strategies to positively impact less happy people. They wanted to answer the question: if you take someone who is unhappy and then you help them to have more social connection, does their happiness improve? While, of course, it is hard to create true social connections such as friendships on someone else's behalf, scientists have done lots of weird and wonderful things to explore what having more human connection does to our happiness.

Nick Epley is one of the scientists who has looked into this.[3] He wanted to see what impact connecting with people during a busy city commute would have on their happiness and to understand what the people involved in the study would predict would happen based on the group they were put into. Now, if you've ever done a city commute on public transport you've probably experienced the eerie quiet between passengers. People tend not to interact, despite being in particularly close proximity to each other. Instead they have their noses buried in books or in their phones, or they're simply in their own world.

Epley conducted an experiment whereby people were put into one of three groups on their way into work on the train. Those in the 'connection group' were asked to have a conversation with a stranger on the train and try to make a meaningful connection; those in the 'solitary group' were asked to enjoy the solitude of their journey and not attempt to interact with others; while those in the 'control group' were asked to do whatever they usually would on their commute. People predicted that they would be most content on their journey if they were put in the solitary group. They thought that they'd be happiest if they didn't have to make an effort with anyone else. The actual results were quite different. The connection group came out the happiest and the least happy group was the solitary group – the ones who'd been asked to keep themselves to themselves and not seek out social connection.

Interestingly, this dynamic of making the wrong prediction when it comes to what we think will make us happy versus what does make us happy is very common. One of the reasons for this dynamic in this study was that people assumed that they would be disturbing someone if they made an attempt to connect. They didn't want to interrupt their thoughts or them reading their book, and so they don't say anything to them at all. But, actually, what the results show is that when we do seek out a social connection, both the person who is trying to connect and the recipient of this connection attempt are far happier than if there is no connection at all.

This is something to keep in mind next time you're on a busy plane or train. In fact, let's think about that for a moment: how do you tend to react when you board a plane? Do you seek out social connection with the person next to you? Or do you tend to politely acknowledge them and then sit in silence for the duration of the flight? What would happen if, next time, you tried to make a positive social connection with them? Try it and see!

Given this research, it's no surprise that building positive relationships is at the centre of the myHappymind system. It's also no surprise that relationships are of critical importance in building your child's happiness and resilience.

As we've seen through these studies, our need for social connection is huge. It would be strange if I didn't mention that I am writing this book during the 2020 coronavirus pandemic, and the narrative that is starting to get louder and louder is around the mental health effects of not having had any social connection with friends or extended family members because of 'lockdown'. There is a reason that solitary confinement is a punishment in prisons! When we starve ourselves of social contact and positive social connection, it negatively affects our mental health and happiness.

Physical presence and happiness

Even the very presence of other people enhances our day-to-day life experiences. One study in 2014 looked at the effect of this during the simple act of eating chocolate.[4] There were just two groups in this study: one was asked to enjoy chocolate with another person, while the other was asked to eat chocolate on their own. The group that enjoyed the chocolate in the company of others rated the experience of eating the chocolate and the taste of the chocolate to be far higher than the other group. This shows us that being with other people and having these shared social connections as we experience life, enhances our overall happiness.

However, it is not the case that any social connection is better than no social connection. It is fair to say that many of us have at some point found ourselves in relationships that no longer serve us positively, for example with a friend. It's quite common for friendships to go through cycles and for there to be times when that friendship is really positive and helps us, and then other times when the friendship no longer serves us. I suspect that you may have already noticed that some of your child's friendships are more positive than others. In fact, sometimes children seem to yearn for those friendships where they are treated less well!

For many of us, we don't spend enough time thinking about and ensuring that the friendships or relationships that we do have are positive and are still bringing us joy. The reality is that the only person in control of our own relationships is us. This is why building positive relationships is such a critical skill as it relates to building our happiness and looking after our mental health. It is also why teaching children how to notice when friendships are positive, or less so, is also incredibly important.

In the next section we'll focus on two key skills that we can use to build positive relationships. These skills are the foundations or building blocks for developing positive relationships and you can start to use them with your child right away. As we review these skills through the lens of your child, I really hope that you'll feel empowered to consider how you use them in your own relationships too. As you now know, it's really important that as a parent you're able to integrate this thinking for yourself before you start to introduce it to your child. This not only allows you to become a better teacher, but it also ensures that you're getting the full benefit from this book.

So, let's dive in and take a look at the first skill that is absolutely critical in building and maintaining positive relationships.

Active Listening

Yes, it really is that simple. The extent to which you are able to be a good listener will have a huge impact on the quality of your relationships. Good listeners make good friends, partners and parents because one of the most fundamental components of a healthy relationship is the ability to communicate, to be heard and to feel heard. As Stephen Covey so brilliantly put it: 'Most people do not listen with the intent to understand; they listen with the intent to reply.'

What he meant by this is that most people when they are listening are doing so through the lens of 'What action do I need to take on the back of this?', rather than thinking, 'What is this person really trying to say to me here?'

When I talk about listening, I'm not just talking about the ability to hear, I'm talking about the ability to listen and really understand where somebody is coming from. It's my view that we have become so busy and so capable of multitasking that we've lost some of the fundamental skills necessary to be good listeners.

In fact, whenever I'm training teachers one of my favourite jokes is to ask: 'Who here has a class full of amazing active listeners?' Nobody responds, but everybody laughs! Because all teachers will tell you that listening is one of the key skills that children need to work on. I don't think this just applies to children either – there are plenty of adults who have a huge opportunity to listen at a deeper level.

Have you ever felt like you're trying to show your feelings, maybe with your partner or a friend, and they're not really listening to you? Like they've not really heard you? How does that make you feel? Frustrated? Lonely? Sad? Not so great, right?

You may also have that friend who is the *best* listener and, after you've poured your heart out to them, you feel so much better, you feel lighter and so grateful. Am I right?

The only difference between the two scenarios that I have just outlined is how effectively the person listened. It may be simple, but it is incredibly impactful. When you develop your active listening skills, you become like that friend who is an amazing listener. You become that person for your partner, your friends and, most importantly, for your child.

Let's take a look at what active listening involves and then we'll see how you'd rate your skills right now. There are several features or skills that characterise a good active listener and they're listed below. (I've included a handy checklist of these in the digital resources – see page 235.)

★ Make eye contact when you're listening to the person who's speaking to you.

★ Show the person that you're listening by nodding your head or smiling so that they can see that you're fully engaged.

★ After they've finished talking, replay what you have heard so that they feel like you've understood them.

★ Ask them questions to clarify what you've heard and ensure that you've interpreted what they're saying correctly.

★ Be fully present – this means no phone, no TV, no radio, just the two of you face to face with no distractions.

If you read this list and thought, crikey, there is a lot to think about here, you're not the only one. But don't worry – you don't have to be actively listening every minute of every day, but you should certainly be tuning into those important moments.

Your active listening skills

Before we begin to look at how to teach these active listening skills to your child, let's take a few moments to reflect on your own active listening skills. Try to see this as a great opportunity for you to really engage with your child. This is something you can practise and improve on so, wherever you are, the only way is up!

Take a few minutes to complete the chart on the next page to review how effectively you actively listen today. As you do this, try to think about yourself in parent mode rather than work or friend mode, as our competence as listeners can change depending on the circumstances we're in. For example, you may feel that you're a brilliant listener when out with a friend for a glass of wine but, actually, as a parent you tend to be so busy when in the house that this is less true. This exercise is for you and no one else – it is to help you grow, so be honest!

How did that feel? How would you rate your active listening skills overall? Give yourself a score out of 10, with 10 being amazing and 1 being that you have significant room for improvement.

If you do have room for growth here, then you're definitely not alone. I cannot tell you how many of the parents I coach have said that just focusing on becoming a better listener with their child or partner has been transformational in their relationships.

Let's review your active listening skills

Skill	100% of the time	Sometimes	Oops! I never do this!
I always make eye contact when I am listening to someone.	☐	☐	☐
I show the person talking that I am listening by nodding my head or smiling.	☐	☐	☐
I replay what they have said to me to show that I have understood them.	☐	☐	☐
I ask them questions to clarify my understanding.	☐	☐	☐
I am fully focused on them, no phone, no TV, all I do is listen.	☐	☐	☐

As you review the chart above, what's the one thing that you're going to commit to doing to improve your active listening skills?

....

....

Your child's active listening skills

Now that we've taken some time to reflect on your listening skills, let's take a look at how effective your child's active listening skills are today. This will help you to consider where to focus. Don't forget that these skills can take time to develop and some children may not be doing any of them right now – this is OK, it is why you are here.

Complete the chart on the next page to explore your child's active listening skills.

What does this tell you about where you have an opportunity to focus on improving your child's active listening skills? Note down these areas of focus below.

....

....

....

....

....

....

Now that we've explored where you and your child are in terms of your active listening skills, let's look at a couple of strategies you can use to build them even further and make this all come to life for your child.

Let's review your child's active listening skills

Skill	100% of the time	Sometimes	Oops! They never do this!
They always make eye contact when they are listening to me.			
They show me that they are listening by nodding their head or smiling.			
They replay what I have said to show that they have understood.			
They ask questions to clarify their understanding.			
They are fully focused on me, no phone, no TV, all they do is listen.			

Listening moments

This is all about creating a dedicated and safe space for your child to talk to you and to feel heard. I suggest getting started by explaining to your child that you are going to start being more intentional about listening to them because you really care about what they have to say. This alone will boost their happiness because you are showing them that they matter.

Then, you can pick a time each day when you will have this listening moment. It may be before bed or over dinner. The timing doesn't matter, but what is important is that you can make this a regular habit and that you can stick to it. Ensure you pick a time when there are no distractions and you can fully focus, so doing this while on the school run is probably not the best idea. You may even decide to merge this with the gratitude habit you've decided on (see pages 117–18).

To start with, just ask them if there is anything they'd like to share, taking the time to practise the active listening skills outlined above. This may be tricky at the start if your child isn't used to it and so some prompts may help, such as:

* How is everything with your friends?
* What are you particularly enjoying at school?
* Is there anything on your mind?

Depending on the age of your child you may need to tweak these prompts or even be a bit more specific, but the trick is to ask an open question and get them talking. Once they start, just practise the active listening skills so that they can see them in action. I can't stress enough how important role modelling is when it comes to teaching active listening.

Next, we'll move into the phase where your child can practise their active listening skills. You can ask your child if they'd like to hear what is on your mind and then use this as an opportunity to share something positive. You may choose to remember an experience that you had together or share a character strength you've noticed them using recently. You'll see here that we are integrating some other parts of the myHappymind system, which can be really powerful. During this segment of your listening moment, you can focus on encouraging your child to practise active listening too. You can remind them to concentrate, ask them to replay what you said or just focus on being in the moment with them. They don't need to know that they are actively listening, but you are teaching them both through modelling it yourself and then prompting them along the way. Don't feel this has to be too rigid though, just keep the active listening skills in mind and use them to guide your approach.

What happens when you instigate a dedicated and special time each day to actively listen without distraction, is that your child learns that they have a safe time and space to share. Rather than carry their worries with them all the time, they know that they can offload them during these listening moments. This helps them to know that they have an opportunity to talk and it makes them feel calmer.

Once your child has established this practice with you at home, they are able to replicate these times with their friends and relationships. They will start to listen more intentionally to their friends and this will help them to build stronger and more meaningful relationships. Starting in the home is the way to embed this first critical relationship-building skill.

I'd like to share an example of how one of the parents in our programme found this strategy to be transformative with her daughter. She knew that her daughter was having a tough time in school as the teachers had flagged this, but she was really struggling to get through to her. Every time she asked her how school was, her daughter would just say 'fine'. When she learnt about active listening, she realised that she was asking her daughter about school as a side thought, when she was distracted doing other things, cooking dinner or trying to clear her inbox – no wonder it wasn't working! So, she decided to implement listening moments with her daughter. At first they talked about lots of things, but her problems at school didn't come up. They stuck with it though and within a few days of regularly putting in place a once-a-day listening moment, her daughter started to open up about what was going on at school. Her mum was amazed and so pleased that her daughter felt able to share. They now do this every night – sometimes they just talk about the best bits of their days (integrating gratitude into this special time), but she knows now that if her daughter needs to, she'll share her worries too.

Role modelling

James Baldwin said in his book *Nobody Knows My Name*: 'Children have never been very good at listening to their elders, but they have never failed to imitate them.' The power of role modelling cannot be underestimated here. When your children see you actively listening to them, guess what happens? They will start listening to you more actively too. Children do what we do, not what we say.

Listening to your child is one of the most critical things you can do for their mental health and ultimately their happiness. When a child feels heard, they feel like they're important and you're teaching them that their feelings matter and so they are more likely to share them with you. As I always say, you are the expert in your own child and you will know when they need to talk to you. The trick is to learn to pick up on the signs and signals that they need to have an important conversation and to practise active listening in those moments.

If your child doesn't feel like they're being heard when they share things with you, even if they seem like little things, they are less likely to share the big things. Let's take the 'after-school chat' that we all like to have with children as an example; we'll often be doing that while making the tea, checking our emails and trying to put a load of washing on at the same time. Can we really listen effectively in that context? The answer, of course, is no.

Understanding Different Perspectives

The second skill which really is a game changer when it comes to building positive relationships is learning to see things from someone else's perspective. This combined with active listening is a powerful tool to forge connections and build and maintain positive relationships.

We often hear about the need to understand, appreciate and embrace diversity as it relates to race, religion or gender. I wholeheartedly agree that this should be part of the fabric of our own self-development as well as something that we consciously address with our children. Here, though, the focus of diversity is slightly different, though no less important. I am talking about the diversity of thought – or of our different perspectives – which is ultimately about diversity of our characters. When we can understand, respect and learn from other people's perspectives, we can build really solid relationships.

Active listening and happiness

Much like expressing gratitude, active listening is a win–win. When you start actively listening with your child over time, you'll notice that they start to do the same.

When you actively listen, the person talking gets dopamine released in their brain and they feel truly connected to you. Because they feel heard and they feel that they matter, they are likely to do the same when it is their turn to listen to you. Then, you'll feel heard, you will feel like you've been listened to and you will get that lovely dopamine release as well. Further to this, it is likely that you will both express gratitude for having listened to each other, which makes you both feel amazing too!

The character strengths tool we met in Chapter 2 (page 85) is a wonderful way to help us to explore other people's perspectives. By using your new knowledge of your own character strengths and those of your child, you can start to think about and consider what other people's strengths may be. This in turn can help you and your child to accelerate the process of understanding other people's perspectives too.

When we don't understand someone's behaviour, we can find it really hard to see their perspective, to empathise, to connect and ultimately to get along with them. Exploring character strengths is so powerful because it gives us a window into the 'why' behind someone's behaviour. It allows us to truly put ourselves in their shoes and start to see why they make the choices that they do in terms of their actions.

Now that you have an understanding of your own character strengths and those of your child, you will be able to start developing the skill of noticing other people's strengths and then seeing the world through their eyes. This will give you and your child the superpower of not only being able to see things from another perspective, but being able to relate to that person and therefore build stronger and more positive relationships with them.

Let me give you an example from a child's perspective of how understanding different character strengths might help us to see things from a different perspective and so strengthen our relationships with others. Let's imagine that this is the first day of school for an eight-year-old boy. He's had to change schools because his parents have moved to a new house. It is break time and he is in the playground on his own looking a bit sad.

A child who has curiosity as their top character strength may go over to him and ask him lots of questions about his last school or his hobbies. The child with humour as a top character strength would probably try to make him laugh by telling him a joke or doing something silly. And the child who has kindness as their top character strength might go over to him and say, 'Are you okay?' or 'Do you want to come and play with us?'

The truth is that each and every one of these children's responses is absolutely OK! They are just different because they all have different character strengths, and it is our strengths that impact how we behave.

If children don't understand the different perspectives and strengths of each other, they may have interpreted each other's actions as being unusual or maybe even inappropriate. The child with kindness as their top strength might think it is really strange that their friend used humour when the new boy is clearly upset; they may think 'this is not the time for jokes!' They may also find it totally bizarre that the child with curiosity was asking him so many questions and think something along the lines of 'give him some space, he obviously doesn't feel like chatting!'

If, though, those children understood their friends' perspectives and were able to notice that each of them was simply using a different character strength, then they wouldn't think this was unusual at all.

You can see how teaching your child to notice other people's character strengths, or even just observe that we all have different character strengths, can be a game changer in terms of how they establish and maintain relationships. This is a unique skill and those who master it are far better at being able to establish and maintain relationships that are built on mutual trust and respect.

Can you relate to this? Have you ever been in a situation where you felt someone else's response seemed strange or even inappropriate? What might this tell you about their character strengths? How, with this new information, can you see this differently?

Your ability to see other perspectives

Before exploring how we can develop this skill with your child, let's first consider the extent to which you're able to notice and see different character strengths in those you spend time with. We're going to start by reminding yourself of your top strengths. Refer back to pages 74–77 and note them down in the space below:

....

....

....

....

....

Now I'd like you to think about your day yesterday. Pick two strengths from the list above and note down how you used them. What did your strengths cause you to think and to do?

....

....

....

....

....

Next, let's think about somebody close to you, perhaps your partner or a friend. Try to pick someone who you think has different strengths to you. Can you note down some of their top strengths? Don't worry about getting the exact language right here, just focus on character rather than competence. Try to come up with three of their strengths and note them below:

....

....

....

How do you see them using these strengths? How do these strengths cause them to behave on a day-to-day basis?

....

....

....

Now, think about a recent interaction with this person — try to pick one where you both had a different response to it. Maybe it was a serious discussion, or you were sharing your feelings about a situation. How did their strengths govern their response?

....

....

....

....

....

In that same interaction, how did your strengths govern your response?

....

....

....

....

....

Hopefully walking through this exercise has helped you to see just how much our strengths govern our responses. We can be faced with the exact same scenario or interaction, but we will often respond to it from a different perspective and this will be largely based on our strengths. As we already know, there are no right or wrong strengths, they are just different. What this means, then, is that the way that you or the other person respond to the interaction we've just discussed isn't right or wrong, it's just different.

When we can start to pause and notice how other people are responding and then tie that back to their character strengths, two things happen:

1. We become more compassionate. Rather than looking at a situation through the lens of right or wrong, we start to look at the situation through the lens of perspective. We become more accommodating to the other person's views.

2. We are better able to build trusting relationships because we are more respectful and understanding of their perspectives. As we learnt earlier, social connection is so important, and we all need to feel valued and heard by others.

When you start to notice other people's strengths and develop an understanding of and compassion for different perspectives, you'll open your mind and become an even stronger relationship builder. This will help you no end, particularly as you learn to tune in to your child's character strengths and perspective. While you may share some character strengths with your child, you will have different perspectives on things and learning to notice this will be a real asset in how you engage and connect with them.

Developing your child's ability to see other perspectives

Before we look at how you can build your child's aware-ness of other perspectives, let's consider the extent to which they already do this. What we're looking for here is whether they're able to see a different point of view which may not be in alignment with their own.

Thinking about simple everyday situations, let's con-sider how they respond when things don't go their way. Perhaps it is deciding what to watch on TV or what to eat for dinner, how do they react when they don't get the out-come that they want?

....

....

....

What does this tell you about where you have an oppor-tunity to support them in understanding other people's perspectives?

....

....

....

What would you do?

This is a really useful, fun and powerful way to teach your child about varying perspectives or points of view.

The idea of this strategy is to explore how different scenarios will create a range of reactions in different people and then to tie this back to character strengths. This approach allows you to help your child to see why people react in different ways and, as a result, develop an understanding of other perspectives – an invaluable tool in building relationships.

To set this up all you need to do is think of a scenario – this can be made up or you can use a real-life example. Having introduced the scenario to your child, you'll just talk about what happened and then explore how different people may react to it. The scenarios you pick with your child will depend on their age, but here is an example so that you can see how this works:

> *You are at the park and you notice a little girl has been waiting for the swings for ages. When it is their turn, another child runs over and gets on the swings first, meaning the little girl has to continue waiting.*

You can simply say to your child, 'What would you do?' As they start to talk about how they would react you can pull out their character strengths. So, for example, if they say, 'I would go over and tell the child who skipped the queue that the little girl was waiting and that wasn't fair', you could notice that this was an example of them using their fairness and bravery strength. Then, you could ask them, 'What might someone else do?' This is where you really start to develop their understanding of other perspectives. You might say, 'If it was me, I would go over and ask the little girl if she was OK' – this would be an example of a kindness strength. The idea is to bring out the point that we all react differently and to then link this back to character strengths.

You may choose to use this strategy when reading a story or watching a film with your child. The scenarios that you discuss are less important than exploring different perspectives so feel free to get creative here! Do remember wherever possible to pull this back to character strengths for maximum impact.

You can use this 'What would you do?' strategy to help your child learn to identify different perspectives. In order for them to be able to consider and respect other perspectives and so build positive relationships, they need to first be able to identify them. By using character strengths as an anchor here we're not only further embedding this tool but we're also addressing this topic from a positive and approachable angle.

By helping your child to see other people's perspectives and character strengths they are also learning empathy – they are learning to walk in another person's shoes and understand them. This is such an important part of building trusting relationships and will support the development of a compassionate child who sees beyond their own needs and wants. This in turn will allow them to establish and maintain positive relationships, and so thrive.

Technology and building relationships

While technology enhances our lives in so many ways, children's increasing use of it means that they are building and maintaining relationships differently. In turn, this means they have far fewer opportunities to use the skills we outlined above because they aren't necessarily having as many moments to connect face to face without distraction.

While it used to be the case that children would spend a lot of face-to-face time with their friends after school and at weekends, it's now more common for them to maintain those relationships via technology, particularly as they get older. Children are playing games together, they're using social media to communicate and it's very hard to use the skills that we've just learnt about while communicating in this way. Practising both active listening and understanding things from another person's perspective are incredibly difficult if we are not physically with that other person.

I'm not saying that children should not be using technology appropriately; it is an incredibly powerful tool and it's not going anywhere. What I am advocating is that, as parents, you consciously think about how they use technology. Getting the balance right between interacting online and ensuring that your child has enough face-to-face time with friends and others to build positive relationships is really important.

While these tools may seem really simple, they're incredibly powerful. Getting into the habit of regularly using both active listening and discussing other perspectives will really help your child to build positive relationships. I cannot emphasise enough the importance of role modelling here too, as so much of our children's 'model' of a good relationship starts with what they see at home.

Now that you've had a chance to reflect on these areas for yourself and for your child, don't be tempted to leave the plan on the pages of this book. It's time to get to work! Remember, these things can take time to develop and so don't be disheartened by that – this is all about taking baby steps forward and starting to impact a change. Teaching children these skills is an investment in their future happiness, don't be tempted to pass it by.

The next chapter will take all of the concepts we've been learning and explore how we can use them in the context of reaching for our dreams. We'll be exploring why dreaming is important for happiness and how it helps to build resilience.

Time to recap

★ There is a direct correlation between the quality of our relationships and our happiness. Social connection is crucial to our well-being – when we have positive social connections with others we feel happier and are better able to cope with life's challenges.

★ Positive relationships make us more resilient as they become like an army of support that forms around and carries us when we're facing tough times. Teaching children how to establish and maintain positive relationships is a critical skill that will serve them throughout life.

★ There are two fundamental relationship-building skills that we can teach children to help them build positive relationships: active listening and understanding different perspectives. Both of these skills take work to establish, but you can get started right away with the tools I have shared and by role modelling at home. Giving these skills to your child is one of the best things you can do to impact their ability to make and sustain positive relationships.

Your digital resources

The key habit that you can get started with immediately and will yield very fast well-being effects is active listening. When you start using active listening with your child you'll see how much more they share with you and you'll feel great about this too. For this chapter, I have given you an active listening poster which you can print out and display somewhere really visible to remind you and your child of the key things to think about when actively listening. This can become a fun way to remind each other and hold each other to account for actively listening – you'll see what I mean when you get started!

See page 235 for details on how to access the digital resources.

My Key Learnings

I want you to use this space to draw, capture and solidify your key reflections from this chapter. What are your 'Aha!' moments and what are you going to do with the learning?

....

....

....

....

....

....

....

....

....

....

....

....

....

....

....

....

CHAPTER 5

Engage: The Power of Goal-setting and Dreaming

'Without dreams and goals there is no living, only merely existing, and that is not why we are here.'

Mark Twain

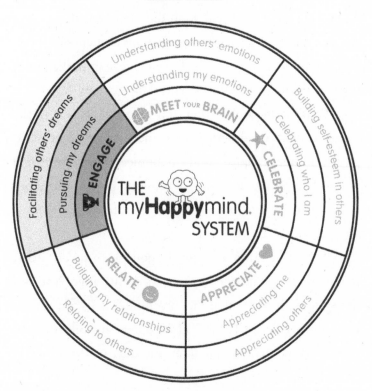

Can we just take a minute to pause and recap on all of the amazing work you've done so far? You've learnt so much and done so much reflection. I am sure by now that you are bursting with ideas about how you can start positively impacting your child's happiness and well-being – and we still have more learning to come!

We've made it to the final part of the myHappymind system which is 'Engage'! This section is focused around the incredible power that accomplishments or achievements have on our happiness and well-being. It also looks at how we can build children's resilience and perseverance through supporting them in setting goals that matter to them.

The reason this is such an important element of the system is that the extent to which we achieve or make things happen in our lives directly correlates to how happy we are. That's why goal-setting and dreaming is one of the simplest and most practical tools that you can employ to positively impact your child's happiness. If we can teach children to get into the habit of thinking proactively about what they want to achieve, then we are giving them a wonderful gift for life.

Here's a question for you: do you like a to-do list? If you're anything like me you're a to-do list ninja! You run your life with lists – you may even have a list for all the lists you need! Am I right? How about this one: do you ever write something on your list that you've actually already done just so you can tick it off? Well, even if you're not guilty of this slightly strange habit, I definitely am!

It might not surprise you that there is in fact a science-based reason that we, as humans, love to set goals and cross things off to-do lists. Our brains love to set goals and to get things done, and they also like to be able to process things in a logical order, which a list allows for. And guess what happens when we actually achieve a goal that is on our list? Yes, that's right – we get that dopamine release in the brain. In fact, even the process of setting a goal and thinking about achieving it releases dopamine. Are you starting to see why we make all of these lists?!

Not All Goals Are Made Equal

Now that we know that setting goals and achieving things is so critical to our happiness, it's time to look at the different types of goals and understand their relative impact as it relates to our well-being.

This is really important because the happiness effect that we get from achieving or thinking about a goal will vary depending on the type of goal. When considering our goals, it's helpful to split them into two broad categories:

1. To-do list goals.
2. Big dream goals.

To-do list goals

Let's talk about our to-do list goals first. These are goals that our circumstances and social constructs set for us. They are things that we need to do because of the many roles that we play in life and our current lifestyle.

Let's look at this from your perspective as an adult first. Whether you are a full-time parent or you have a job alongside looking after your family, you have a lot of things that you have to do. Your situational context leads to the setting of the majority of your goals.

In terms of our domestic and parenting to-do list goals, these include the weekly food shop, paying bills, organising family events and play dates, etc. And, at work, your job will give you a set of objectives or things that you need to complete in order to fulfil your specific role.

In terms of our children's to-do list goals, they tend to be set either by us as parents or by their teachers. At home they may have goals, such as keeping their bedroom tidy or clearing their plate after dinner. At school they may be set goals like learning their spellings or reading a book. While none of us would argue with any of these goals because they're all perfectly reasonable, they are all in this to-do list category. They are things that we just need to get done.

Can you see how life just gives us a lot of activity or goals that we need to complete in order to fulfil our day-to-day responsibilities?

Big dream goals

On the other side of the spectrum are big dream goals. These are goals or things that we personally want to achieve. They are based on our passions and are things that we have dreamt of making happen. If you're a runner, you may have a goal of running your first marathon. Or maybe you've always wanted to start your own business or write a book. Whatever these goals are for you, they are things that you are super passionate about achieving.

From a child's perspective, they may dream of building a particular Lego structure or of being able to develop a certain dance move. Even from the youngest of ages, children start to develop their dreams and passions. These aren't things that need to happen in order for them to do well at school or be well-behaved at home; they are things that they *love* and deeply care about achieving.

The science of goal-setting

The research shows us that thinking about goals in very specific ways gives us a much greater chance of achieving them. This is why it is so important that you really consider what success looks like. 'Goal specificity' is a term often used to describe this. When we can be really specific about our goals and apply some quantitative specificity to them, the likelihood of us achieving them increases. Psychologist Howard Klein and his colleagues carried out a study where they asked the students in a hand-eye coordination test whether they had a specific performance goal.[1] Those who did performed so much better in the test than those who didn't because they had a really specific strategy. Having a quantitative performance target ensures you make a plan and then you're likely to perform better.

Further, when you think about your goal and what the outcome will look like in a really detailed way, this helps you to achieve it. But, alongside this, we have to also think through the obstacles that might get in our way and consider how we will overcome them. Scientists call this 'mental contrasting' and it is a visualisation technique that involves thinking about the positive outcome and then thinking about obstacles that might get in the way of us achieving it.

Thinking about both the positive outcome that we want and the challenges that we may face to get there hugely impacts our likelihood of achieving our goal. This is because when we've considered the potential obstacles that we might face we're more likely to plan for them and so overcome them.

Gertraud Stadler of Columbia University performed a study looking at the impact of this mental contrasting technique involving getting women to work towards eating more fruit and vegetables.[2] She found that if they used this mental contrasting technique and considered the downside of not getting healthy as well as the upside of it, they sustained the habit of healthy eating for much longer. If they just thought about the upside, they still saw an improvement in their eating, but the habit didn't last as long.

Assessing Your Goals

The types of goals or accomplishments that give us the greatest well-being effect are our big dream goals, or those goals that we've really dreamt of or aspired to.

It is the achievement of these goals that gives us the big dopamine release in our brains. In fact, even recalling the memory of a big dream accomplishment gives us a well-being boost. So, if you had dreamt of completing a marathon and you do so, thinking back to crossing the finish line will give you a dopamine release – even years later! The bigger the aspiration and the more passionate we are about the goal, the bigger the well-being effect we receive.

That's not to say that you don't get any well-being effect from clearing your to-do list goals – you absolutely do – but it is less of a happiness boost than when you achieve those big dream goals. When you clear your ironing basket or get the shopping put away or submit that report at work, you will still benefit from the sense of achievement (and get that happiness boost), but just not to the same extent as when you finish that marathon.

This seems obvious right? The more we want to achieve something, the bigger the happiness effect when we do.

But let me ask you this: where do you spend most of your time and effort? Is it on your to-do list goals or on your big dream goals?

If you're able to say that you are fully focused on spending your time on fulfilling your big dream goals then, congratulations! However, I'm pretty sure that for most of us we feel that there's an opportunity to spend more time focusing on those things that we really want to achieve – on our big dream goals.

In fact, the majority of parents in my programme tell me that they are desperate to get a better balance between their to-do lists goals and their big dream goals. This is something that I wholeheartedly encourage because, as we know, it will have a direct and positive impact on our happiness.

Before we start to look at how you can support your child in defining and working towards their big dream goals, let's see where you fall on the spectrum of prioritising your big dreams versus your to-do list goals. I'd like you to complete the following exercise – again, this is for you so just go with it and be honest.

What proportion of your goals would you say are to-do list goals i.e. things that you just have to get done because of your role or your work, versus your big dream goals i.e. things that you really dream and aspire to and want to achieve? Maybe think of this as a ratio: is it 80:20, 60:40, 20:80?

....

....

....

What does this tell you? Do you feel like you're focused on the right areas or is there room for some adjustment?

Our to-do list goals can often leave us so busy and exhausted(!) that we forget about setting our big dreams and aspirations. And while, of course, there are things that we just need to make happen, we can always find time to pursue our passions and, as we've seen, this has huge well-being benefits.

Given what we know about how much our big dream goals can positively affect our happiness, I'd like you to consider how you can ensure you're encompassing them into your life as an adult. If you feel like you aren't spending enough time here, why not try to carve out a time each week that is dedicated to you pursuing your big dream goals? Maybe it is a Saturday morning where you ringfence a couple of hours to work on them. We'll look at what it takes to set and achieve goals in the next section, but I really encourage you to apply this for yourself as well as your child. Not only will this positively impact your well-being, but you'll be role modelling this to your child too.

How to Set Big Dream Goals
with Your Child

'A goal without a plan is just a wish.'
Antoine de Saint-Exupéry, *The Little Prince*

The well-being effect from achieving our big dream goals applies as much to our children as it does to us. So, it is critical that from a young age we're inspiring children with the ability and the desire to set their own goals. If we don't proactively do this, the risk is that they believe that they should only be focused on achieving those things that others ask of them, whether this is us as parents or their teachers. Again, of course, these things *are* important, but we also want them to have big dreams and aspirations, and if we can start this young, they'll develop this as a habit of a lifetime.

So, how do you get your child to start setting and working towards their big dream goals? Well, it all starts with noticing their passions and then helping them to set a goal. Helping your child to come up with a goal might be really easy for you if they have an existing hobby, but what if you're not so sure? The way to tackle this is just to observe where they spend their free time; what do they get up to when they're totally relaxed? Noticing this will really help you to spot where they have a passion and therefore what goals they might want to set. Maybe you've seen them trying to build a really tall Lego tower or you've noticed them practising a trick on their bike over and over again. The key thing here is that, whatever the big dream goal is, it has to be something that your child is *really* passionate about. This is not about what we want them to achieve, it is about helping them to uncover their own aspirations.

> One of the parents in our programme felt like her son had no hobbies and so was really struggling to come up with a goal. She watched and noticed where he was spending his time and realised that he was constantly doodling and trying to draw a dinosaur. When she observed this and they talked about it, she realised this was the right place to focus. Together they set the goal of him being able to draw a T-Rex and they were off!

Once you are clear on a goal that your child is passionate about, you can use my five-step framework to help them get there. Let's walk through this framework which draws on what we know about effective goal-setting. We'll use a real example of a child's goal so that you can see how powerful it is. The child's big dream goal is to learn how to play the piano.

Step 1: Define what you want to achieve

Make this as specific as you can and attach a numerical value to it if possible so that there is a definitive moment when your child knows they have achieved it.

Child example: 'I will complete my Grade 1 piano exam by September next year.'

Top tip: Your child may need help here to make this specific. By just talking to them about their goal you'll be able to support them in making it really clear.

Step 2: Define what success will look like

How will they know when they have achieved their goal? Support your child in trying to really visualise this and again make it very specific. What measures can they put in place so that they know they've achieved it? How will they feel?

Child example: 'I will be able to play five different pieces on the piano and I will feel so proud of myself that I can read music. I will hang my Grade 1 certificate on the wall in my bedroom.'

Top tip: The more you can encourage your child to imagine their success here the better. Using prompts like, 'What will you see when you have achieved it and how will you feel?' can be really helpful.

Step 3: What help will you need to achieve it?

This is a critical step. Do they need support from someone? Do you need to invest in something for them? This might be resources, people, new learning, etc. Really think this one through so that you have identified all the help they need.

Child example: 'I will need help from a piano teacher and I will need my parents to buy me piano books.'

Top tip: As you are helping your child to think through what help they need, you can use this as an opportunity to reflect on gratitude and also to help them get comfortable with accepting help.

Step 4: What obstacles might you face? How will you overcome them?

This may seem unusual but, as we learnt earlier, thinking through potential obstacles and having a plan to overcome them is often the key differentiator between achieving our goals and not.

Child example: 'I might be too busy and tired to practise with all of my other after-school commitments and so I need to prioritise practising piano.'

Top tip: Help your child to get comfortable with thinking about what obstacles they may face and encourage them so that they understand this is normal and that they can overcome them. This really helps to avoid them 'giving up' at the first hurdle and to develop perseverance.

Step 5: How will you celebrate when you achieve it?

What will you do to mark their success? Again, be specific.

Child example: 'I will invite my grandparents over for a piano concert and then we'll go to my favourite restaurant for dinner.'

Top tip: It is important that your child defines the celebration – let them be the one to pick what they do to mark their achievement (within reason!).

Using this framework to help your child think through and plan out their goals will help them to become more intentional about what they are trying to achieve. It will also supercharge their chances of getting there and provide a real source of structure and motivation for them. Making sure that we dedicate time to allow children the space to pursue their big dream goals is really important. Sometimes life gets so packed full of activities and to-do list goals that children don't have the space to pursue their dreams – this is something that as parents we should be mindful of to ensure the balance is right.

How to Teach Perseverance

As well as the big well-being effects that setting big dream goals brings, helping your child to work towards their goals develops their resilience and perseverance.

Thomas Edison said: 'Many of life's failures are people who did not realise how close they were to success when they gave up.' Perseverance is one of the most critical skills to teach children. If they can persevere when they are faced with challenges, not only will they achieve more but they'll learn to cope with difficulties and knockbacks more effectively too.

A lot of the parents I coach tell me this is one of their big 'Aha!' moments when they take our courses. When and where we focus on helping our children to persevere can have such a transformational impact on whether they develop their resilience muscle or not.

Most of the time, when we're talking to children about needing to just keep going or to persevere, we're doing so about areas or tasks that they find challenging. Whether that's maths or music or sport, our dialogue around perseverance is often most prevalent in those areas in which our children struggle.

Let's just note down what those areas might be for your child below. Where do you tend to focus your perseverance conversations with them?

....

....

....

What do you notice about when your conversations around perseverance tend to happen? Are they focused around where your child's passions lie? Or do you tend to talk about persevering when they are working on something that they are not that interested in?

....

....

....

You may well have found that you've come up against some resistance from your child when you've encouraged them to persevere. Maybe they've felt that they 'just can't do it' or that they'll 'never get it done' (we'll talk more about that in the next chapter). One thing's for sure, it isn't always easy to teach children perseverance.

Focus on your child's big dream goals

Given we all want to teach our children to be able to persevere when times get tough, it's fair to assume that we want to make it as easy as possible for them to learn this skill, right? So, what might happen if rather than focusing our perseverance efforts around those things that our children struggle with, we focused them around those areas that they are passionate about?

I'll say this again because it is so important: teaching perseverance is so much easier when you are doing so in the context of something your child is passionate about achieving (their big dream goals) than when you're focused on an area that they're not passionate about (to-do list goals).

Let's explore this further. Take, for example, a little girl who struggles with learning her eight times table but who is football crazy and desperate to achieve doing 20 keepy-uppies (for non-UK readers this is a trick where you keep the football up in the air by kicking it with your foot without letting it touch the floor). Which goal do you think she will be most motivated to achieve? Mastering her eight times table or doing 20 keepy-uppies?

You guessed it – the keepy-uppies! She will be so determined to achieve this goal because it is something that *she* cares about rather than something that she just has to do, and so she'll show far more persistence and perseverance.

In turn, when she achieves this goal, she'll get a huge well-being benefit because she really cares about it. In contrast she might be happy when she finally learns that eight times table (because she won't need to practise it anymore!), but she won't get the same well-being effect as she will from achieving the keepy-uppies.

When children set their goals based on their big dream goals rather than their to-do list goals, their motivation to achieve them goes through the roof and they will persevere!

Of course, children need to understand that there are things in life that they just need to achieve, like their to-do list goals. However, they also need to understand and learn how to set passion-led goals based on their own desires and dreams. Teaching them how to do this using my five-step framework is a gift that keeps on giving because it helps children to believe that they have the power and the ability to achieve whatever they desire. While at first they'll need to use the framework with you to get the hang of it, once they see it working they'll use it on autopilot. When I speak to my son now about achieving a goal, he uses the framework without even realising it – he considers all the steps, including the potential roadblocks and what he wants to do to celebrate when he achieves it. This has just become part of how he thinks.

This approach of focusing on passion-led goals to demonstrate and teach perseverance is particularly important if your child lacks the self-confidence to keep going when they struggle with something. If that something is a to-do list goal, or something that they're not necessarily that passionate about *and* they don't really believe that they can achieve it, this can be an uphill battle.

In this situation, a teacher or parent may say things like, 'Come on, you can do it, you just need to practise.' But, here's the rub, if this child doesn't believe that they can ever achieve it then words like this just have no meaning. In fact, they can often serve to demotivate the child instead.

This is why using big dream goals to help your child to learn perseverance is so powerful.

Give your child their own evidence

Often children won't persevere with something because they fundamentally believe that they cannot do hard things or that, even if they keep trying, they'll never get there.

As parents we often spend hours willing them on, encouraging them and telling them that 'we believe in them'. The fact is this: children need to see their own evidence to believe in themselves. The best strategy when a child is struggling with something is to give them their own evidence that they do have the skill of perseverance and that they can achieve things when they keep trying.

We must help them to see this evidence not through something that they are struggling with, but instead through something that they love and are passionate about. Let's go back to the keepy-uppy example – that little girl will practise for hours to accomplish her goal because she's so passionate about it, right? By celebrating her perseverance as she practises, we're reminding her that she can persevere. Then, when she faces something that she finds less easy like that eight times table, we can remind her that she has the skill of perseverance because she used it when learning to do the keepy-uppies. Rather than us just telling her that she can do it, we are showing her that she has the skill of perseverance and that she used it with the keepy-uppies so she can use it with the times table too.

Can you see how we're building resilience by focusing on the child's passion rather than something that they don't have that much interest in? Once again, by using positive psychology components and focusing on the child's strengths rather than on the things that perhaps come less naturally, we're able to help build their confidence, self-esteem and, ultimately, their resilience.

This is why goal-setting is so important. It is not just about the general well-being effect that children will get from setting and achieving goals. It is also about building their perseverance skills and their resilience.

When children set big dream goals that they're passionate about, they'll keep going even when they fail. When children set goals that they're passionate about, they'll get up again when they fall over. And when children set goals that they're passionate about, you'll see the true might of their perseverance.

In contrast, if a child is only ever asked to focus on those things that we as parents or teachers want them to achieve, this looks very different. Therefore, I encourage you as parents to use goal-setting with your child as much as possible but let these goals be led by their passions and dreams.

Engage: The Power of Goal-setting and Dreaming

Let school be the place where to-do list goals get set for your child, and let your focus be on helping them to learn the skill of setting big dream goals. For when we teach a child to dream, we give them wings.

Setting Your Big Dream Goals

This next section is dedicated to thinking about how we can shift the balance so that *you're* better able to pursue those goals that are in alignment with your dreams, alongside being focused on your to-do list goals. This is important for all of the happiness benefits we've explored, but also because one of the most powerful ways to get your child to focus on their big dream goals is to see you doing it!

We're going to take a look at your approach to goal-setting today and see where you might have opportunities moving forward to further align this with my five-step framework.

Using the space below, note down how you set goals today. Do you do this in a structured way? Or do you just think about them in your head?

....

....

....

Do you have any big dream goals that you've been thinking about doing for a long time, but for whatever reason you've just not got round to them? Write them down in the space below.

....

....

....

What you may have found in going through this exercise is that, firstly, you don't necessarily have a really structured approach to goal-setting (don't worry, we're about to change that). You may have also noticed that, as you start to actively think about it, there are lots of things you'd like to achieve that you just never seem to have time for.

If this resonates (which it does for most parents!), I'd like you to use this as an opportunity or a moment in time where you vow to change that. I'm going to ask you to think about which one of those big dream goals you're going to start actively pursuing. It's important to use a real example to get the most out of this exercise and, remember, you doing this allows you to better coach your child when you start helping them to set their big dream goals.

Looking at the list of things you've been wanting to achieve but just haven't got round to, pick one of them. I'd like you to choose something that is a short- to medium-term goal, so it's going to take between two and four weeks to complete. Make sure that this is genuinely a goal that you're passionate about, so it isn't cleaning the driveway or sorting out the kids' clothes, unless you're particularly passionate about those things, of course! Maybe for you it is reading that book that you were given at Christmas or you want to join a Pilates class.

Having chosen the goal, we're going to use my five-step process for planning it out (see page 177 for more details). As we've already seen, this approach encompasses the things that matter most when it comes to setting goals.

Step 1: Define what you want to achieve
Make this as specific as you can. Rather than saying: 'I want to join a Pilates class', you might say: 'I will do at least two Pilates classes a week for the next four weeks.'

....

....

....

Step 2: Define what success will look like
How will you know when you have achieved your goal?

....

....

....

Step 3: What help will you need to achieve it?

Do you need support from a partner? Do you need to invest in something?

....

....

....

Step 4: What obstacles might you face? How will you overcome them?

Think through potential obstacles and have a plan to overcome them.

....

....

....

Step 5: How will you celebrate when you achieve it?

What will you do to mark your success?

....

....

....

For those of you who've completed this process fully – congratulations! I hope that you can feel the impact that actually thinking through and planning out your goal has had on your belief that you can achieve it. I'm willing to bet that you already feel more motivated and more excited about getting started in pursuing this goal than you did before.

Having been through this process, I'm sure you can see why it's so important to dedicate some mental space to thinking about what we want to achieve and then to plan it out, unlike our to-do list goals, which have a habit of being very top of mind and often in our face! Our desire to achieve our big dreams may be huge, but they often just slip down the priority list. This is why planning out our goals is such a critical skill for us to master and to teach to our children.

The good news is that you've made it all the way to the end of the book and so you've done what can often be the hardest part of any change – you've started! I hope I've given you lots to think about and lots to start reflecting on. Now it's time to take what you've learnt and start figuring out which parts of the system you feel are going to be most powerful for you and your child, and to get started.

Time to recap

★ Goal-setting is a key component of the myHappymind system because accomplishment or getting things done has a huge impact on our happiness and well-being. Quite simply, those of us who get things done or make things happen are happier than those of us who don't.

⋆ It's so easy to get caught up in just 'doing' all of the time that we forget how to dream, or we never learn in the first place. Focusing on our big dreams is where we see the biggest well-being benefits and so it's important to have a balance between our to-do list goals and those that we're really passionate about.

⋆ My five-step framework for setting goals maximises the chances of you and your child achieving them (see page 177). This framework draws on the robust science and research that shows that taking time to plan, visualise and prepare for our goals massively impacts our chances of success. You can use this with your child, as well as for your own goals.

⋆ As parents we need to ensure that our children don't become so bogged down in their day-to-day goals or chores that they fail to set big dream goals. This is not just important for their well-being but also because these big dream goals are an incredibly powerful way to teach perseverance. When children learn to persevere, they're able to conquer the world, but we have to show them that they can do this.

Engage: The Power of Goal-setting and Dreaming

Your digital resources

One of the key things that will supercharge your child's (and your own) goal-setting ability is learning how to set goals in a way that all of those research-backed techniques show us work! This is why I'm giving you a goal-setting template as your digital resource. You can download this template and print it out each time you or your child is putting in place a goal. This will help them, and you, ensure you're considering all of the areas that matter when it comes to setting meaningful and impactful goals.

See page 235 for details on how to access the digital resources.

My Key Learnings

I want you to use this space to draw, capture and solidify your key reflections from this chapter. What are your 'Aha!' moments and what are you going to do with the learning?

....

....

....

....

....

....

....

....

....

....

....

....

....

....

....

....

....

....

CHAPTER 6
Putting It All Together

'There are only two mistakes one can make along the
road to truth; not going all the way, and not starting.'
Buddha

At the beginning of this book I spoke at length about overwhelm, and we discussed the fact that it can come on when we are seeking change. I want you to know that if you are feeling any sense of overwhelm in terms of where to begin that is absolutely to be expected. In fact, it is a sign that you're already starting to grow because your brain is beginning to process all that you've learnt and consider how to make it stick.

Those feelings of growth and change can present themselves in different ways and this can be a time when those stories we talked about right at the beginning can start coming up again. Stories like: 'This all makes total sense, but, really, I just don't think my kids will ever start sharing gratitude' or 'There is no way my child will ever take to happy breathing' or 'I am just too busy to introduce any of this into my life right now.'

All of these stories are a way for our brain to resist change. We resist change because it threatens our habits and our normal way of doing things – it takes us away from our comfort zone. In his book, *Unleash the Power Within* Tony Robbins said: 'All growth starts at the end of your comfort zone' and this is true for all aspects of our life, including changing the way we look after the mental health of ourselves and our children.

Let's keep it real here and acknowledge what some of these thoughts or stories might be for you. Are they about time or your ability to introduce this to your family? Note them all down here – this can be an incredibly powerful way to acknowledge them before we move on and focus on how we can and will implement some changes.

....

....

....

....

....

Now you've captured those thoughts, we can look at them from afar and recognise this: thoughts aren't facts. Just because we are thinking them, it doesn't make them true. This practice of noticing your thoughts and acknowledging that they are just thoughts and that they aren't true is an incredibly important part of this journey. In fact, it is a skill which, if you can master it, will change so many aspects of your life.

Remember in Chapter 1 we explored how our thoughts lead to our feelings and then our feelings lead to our behaviours and actions (page 44)? You can see that if you allow negative thoughts to take hold, they're going to influence your feelings and behaviours. Ultimately, they are going to be responsible for the outcomes that you achieve. In order to move forward positively and with the most impact, I want to show you how you can shift your thoughts with a really simple strategy.

In the space below I want you to write three positive statements or thoughts that you have about what you've learnt and how you'll take it forward. For example, 'I can implement a gratitude habit' or 'I will start to set big dream goals with my child.'

....

....

....

....

....

Now, humour me for a minute here – I want you to just read over them a few times and really start to believe them. When we start to pay attention to our thoughts in this way, we're able to shift them, which will then impact our feelings (I bet you're feeling more positive about this already?!), and then that will impact your behaviour. Come back to these statements whenever you're feeling overwhelmed or like it's all too much because it's likely that if you're feeling that, those negative thoughts have taken hold again.

Now that we've got you in a positive frame of mind about how you'll implement the strategies you've learnt throughout this book, we're going to get laser focused on where the myHappymind system can best help you and your family. First, though, I want to spend some time talking about the incredible power of habits. When we better understand how our brains work and what happens when we learn, you'll see how setting up some regular routines with your family around the system is well within your reach. I've said it before, and I'll say it again – you've got this!

Let's go back to some science and learn about how our brains learn and create habits.

Our Brains and Habits

'Motivation is what gets you started. Habits is what keeps you going.'
Jim Rhon, *The Five Major Pieces of the Life Puzzle*

I hope by now that you are feeling motivated to get going and start making the shifts that we've talked about to build your child's resilience, confidence and self-esteem. You were motivated to buy this book, you've been motivated to read it up to here and now you're motivated to make some changes because you can see how important it is. All of that is wonderful, and it serves as the kick-start to get you going, but in order for what you've learnt to have a true and lasting impact, we have to turn them into habits.

If we take gratitude as an example, I'm sure you may have already started to express more gratitude to your child and those around you, and that is amazing. But let me be honest with you for a second, we often start something but don't quite manage to make it stick as a habit. We get busy, we fall into our old ways and we forget to do the things that we promised ourselves we'd do. Have you ever decided you are absolutely going to start something – like reading every night before bed or not working late anymore – and you stick at it for a few days and then *life* happens?! You get so busy sorting out the kids and the house that you just don't have the energy to read. Or you just have to get through this one deadline at work and then you'll stop pulling the late-nighters. Any of this feeling familiar?

We've all done this and it's what makes us human. However, I want you to make a promise to yourself that with the habits we're going to create around looking after your entire family's mental health, you won't let that happen. Because we're going to do the work now to ensure that you understand how habits are formed, and I am going to introduce you to some clever hacks that will ensure that you stick with them.

Let's make a start by talking about what happens in our brains when we learn and then we'll dive into habits. The reason I want to explain these two things it that when we understand the science, it really helps us to make things stick. This isn't some fluffy concept – it is real, hard science.

The science of habits

One of the first stages of introducing a new habit is ensuring we feel comfortable with how to do the task or the act itself. Let's take goal-setting as an example. If you haven't used a structured process like my five-step framework on pages 177–81, then it may take a few times to get the hang of setting a goal in this way. But, when you've done it a few times, it'll become easier and easier. This is because of a concept called 'neuroplasticity'. Neuroplasticity refers to the brain's ability to adapt or, as neuropsychologist Dr Celeste Campbell puts it: 'It refers to the physiological changes in the brain that happen as the result of our interactions with our environment. From the time the brain begins to develop in utero until the day we die, the connections among the cells in our brains reorganize in response to our changing needs. This dynamic process allows us to learn from and adapt to different experiences.'[1]

Putting It All Together

In essence, neuroplasticity is the process that happens in our brains when we learn and grow. But how exactly does it do this? Our brains are made up of millions and millions of cells called neurons. A neuron's prime function is to send messages around our brain and, when they do this, something called a neural pathway gets created. If, for example, I was reaching to pick up a piece of fruit from the fruit basket, the neurons will be sending messages to each other to allow me to perform that function. In that process a neural pathway gets formed – these neural pathways are links between neurons that 'wire' the brain so that the brain can control different body functions and thinking processes.

This process of the brain growing and the brain remembering based on those neural pathways that have built up is called neuroplasticity. The key thing to remember here is that when we practise something over and over again, the neural pathways get stronger and stronger until such a time when that activity or that function becomes something that we can do on autopilot.

Let's take the example of your child learning to ride a bike. The first time they try, it feels so hard – almost unachievable. They're wobbling all over the place, they can't coordinate their arms and legs, they're not sure what they should be doing and they're petrified that they'll fall. But each time they practise, those neural pathways get stronger. They remember the different things that they need to do with their body to ride the bike and the brain remembers. And then the next time they get on the bike it's a little bit easier, they're not quite as wobbly, and so on and so forth, until they can ride their bike. The neural pathway has become so strong that they don't even need to think about it.

In fact, we can go for years without riding a bike and then get back on it and off we go – this is because those neural pathways are still there. This is neuroplasticity in action. Once we've established those neural pathways, they stay with us and things are so much easier, but we do have to put the work in at the start to establish them.

How do I get started?

Do you want to know the best way to get started with implementing a new habit? Just get started! It really is that simple. The first step to truly integrating these strategies into your family life is to just begin taking action. Start using the strategies you've learnt with your child and, even if they feel strange or not in sync with what you'd usually do as a family, keep going with them. Neuroplasticity will help you to make these things come more naturally with time, but it does require you and your child to put the effort in first.

If you and your child can practise the strategies we've learnt about in the book over and over again, with time your brains will remember and grow through this process of neuroplasticity. Then you can both start to turn them into habits and just do them on autopilot. This is when they'll really help your child in developing resilience, self-esteem and happiness, now and for a lifetime.

Explaining neuroplasticity to your child

I want to share with you a really simple exercise to help your child understand the concept of neuroplasticity because it will help them in engaging with these habits and in their learning in general. This exercise is based on one of the exercises we do in our programme and is focused around writing. You may need to tweak this depending on the age of your child, but you can do this with most ages if they can hold and make some kind of shape with a pencil:

1. Ask your child to write a really simple sentence (or draw a shape if they are younger); for example, 'Hello my name is . . .' Ask them to do this with their normal writing hand.
2. After they've written that sentence, simply ask them, 'How did you find that?' And they're likely to say, 'It was easy' or 'It was fine.'

3. Then ask them, 'What do you notice about your writing?' and they're likely to say something like, 'It looks like it always does.'

4. Next, ask them to write the same sentence or draw the same shape but with their non-writing hand.

5. After they've written the sentence or drawn the shape, ask them 'How was that?' They're likely to say 'It was harder' or 'My writing isn't as neat.'

What you're doing here is helping your child to see that writing with their normal writing hand (because they've done that over and over and over again) is much easier than writing with their non-writing hand. The reason for this is because the neural pathways have become so strong in their normal writing hand. However, they haven't yet developed the same neural pathways in their other hand because they haven't practised as much. Of course, if they were to practise writing with their other hand, over time that would become easier, too.

Finding ways to make this relevant for children and using real examples that they can relate to is really helpful. If your child really struggled to learn how to catch a ball, that would be a great example to use too. You could say to them something like, 'Do you remember when you could never catch that ball, but you practised and practised, and your neural pathways formed and now it's easy for you?'

Maybe it's algebra for your child or learning to ride their bike. It doesn't matter what you choose, the point is that you find examples that will resonate for your child. Just like we explored with perseverance, we want to show them their own evidence that they have already used neuroplasticity, so they can absolutely use it again.

Neuroplasticity puts some science behind the phrase 'practice makes perfect'. For some children, saying things like this to them can actually have the opposite effect. If a child doesn't believe in themselves or they have low self-esteem, it can actually be quite demotivating to be told that 'practice makes perfect' because, fundamentally, they don't believe that they can ever achieve the things they're working towards.

However, when they understand the science and the concept of neuroplasticity, they start to believe that they can get better at something. Children tend to interpret science as fact, which is why bringing science to them is so powerful in helping them to understand how they can grow and develop.

The Amazing Power of Habits

Habits are so fascinating. We all have a ton of them and sometimes they're positive and sometimes, well, less so! Often, though, we don't even realise that something is a habit – it is so engrained in who we are and what we do that we don't even notice that it is there.

For example, how do you make your cup of tea or coffee? I bet you have a set routine: you pick your mug, then you boil the kettle, or do you boil the kettle and then pick your mug? Next, you might put the tea bag in your cup and add the sugar, or does the sugar go in first? We all do this same simple task differently, but get the same result at the end, but it's our habits that determine *how* we do it. We are very unlikely to do it differently each time because we are just operating on autopilot – this is a great example of a habit that we have but that we're not necessarily aware of, until now! You'll have hundreds of habits just like this, and the more you think about them, the more you'll spot them.

Let's start by just noting down some of your positive habits and some of your less positive habits:

Positive habits:

....

....

....

....

....

Less positive habits:

....

....

....

....

....

You may have noticed some things here that you're really happy about in terms of your positive habits and some things that you're less proud of, your negative habits. The good news is that you can change these habits and start to build some new ones, and neuroplasticity will really help you to make this happen.

Aristotle said, 'We are what we repeatedly do. Excellence, then, is not an act, but a habit.' This is such a beautiful quote because the only way that we get brilliant at anything is through practice, by keeping going and building those neural pathways. We're looking to help our children understand that we are the product of our choices and what we do and that, if we're motivated enough to put the work and practice in over and over again, we can achieve amazing things.

Excellence is not something that we're born with; it is achieved by forming positive habits and sticking with them.

How to Make Habits Stick

We all know the importance of persistence and consistency when it comes to building a habit – that goes without saying. So, why is it still so hard to implement a new habit?

How many times have you started a new regime or habit, whether it's a diet or a training programme, and you fell off the wagon in the first week? I know I am guilty of this! We've all been there and that's because it's really, really hard in the beginning to establish those new neural pathways. We are also competing against those unhelpful thoughts going around in our head which, as we've seen, then impact our feelings and behaviours. Ultimately our brains don't like change and so we have to push through that initial resistance and get used to it by building those neural pathways, then it becomes a breeze!

We're going to look at two really helpful strategies that science has shown help us to turn our positive intentions into habits that stick.

Situational support

The first strategy we're going to look at is called 'situational support'. This refers to the situation and how it can serve to either help or hinder us as we try to establish a habit.

Let's take the example of healthy eating. You've decided that you want to stop snacking on chocolate and crisps and start eating more healthy foods like fruit and vegetables. Here is how the situation might affect this: if we were to clear out our cupboards of all those unhealthy snacks and instead prepare lots of ready-to-eat fruit and vegetables in the fridge, guess what? We're more likely to stick to it because we've controlled our environment in such a way that there are no unhealthy snacks in the house and healthy snacks are readily available. We've created a situation whereby it is easier to stick to our habit and, as a result, we're more likely to be successful. In turn, those neural pathways will form more easily and we'll get into the habit sooner.

There are some really robust studies that affirm the importance of creating the right situations in order to help us stick to our habits or new intentions. Let's take a look at one of those studies now.

Professor and researcher Brian Wansink and his colleagues carried out some research into how the situation can affect our behaviour.[2] He found that this kind of situational support is even more powerful than willpower as it relates to changing our behaviour. He conducted a study in an office environment to see how the location of a bowl of treats impacted how many treats people would eat.

For the first group, the bowl of treats was placed in a highly visible place on the desk and for the second group the bowl of treats was placed two metres away from the desk. The study found that when the treats were on the desk the group consumed 48 per cent more of them than when they were two metres away, and that visibility of the treats made a difference to consumption – when the treats were placed inside the desk drawer, people consumed 25 per cent fewer than when they were on top of the desk. This tells us that both the visibility of something and the convenience of accessing it or its location hugely affect our behaviour. So how can we use this to our advantage?

We know that the situation that we create around the habit that we are trying to instil has a huge impact on our likelihood of following through with it. If you're determined to instil a gratitude habit on the back of what you've learnt in the book, you could invest in a journal which you have on your bedside table to remind you to capture what you're grateful for each day. Or, you could make dinner time the time when you discuss gratitude with your child and make a little 'Gratitude Time' sign with them.

One of the reasons I have given you some posters as part of your digital resources is because, by being able to see Team HAP or the active listening checklist for example, you are more likely to remember to integrate these concepts into the conversations you have and the approaches you take with your child. Likewise, by giving you an audio file of the happy breathing exercise, you can get started right away. By making this easy to access, I am increasing your chances of actually using it and, in turn, increasing your chances of being able to establish that as a habit with your child.

These things might sound silly and small, but they are actually hugely powerful, and they work. When we see something that will remind us to engage in the positive habit, we are far more likely to actually complete it. Here is an example of how I have used situational support with my son. We used to battle over him getting dressed for school as soon as he woke up rather than coming downstairs in his pyjamas and putting the TV on. To shift this and create a habit where he just puts his uniform on as soon as he wakes up, I started laying out his uniform the night before in front of his door. The visibility and ease of access to the uniform meant he would put it straight on (he had to step over it to leave the room!). Now it is the first thing he does on a school day and, so, no more nagging!

Accountability partners

The second strategy we can use to help us make those habits stick is to ensure we have an accountability partner, or that we make our habit known and social. Since we are fundamentally social creatures and we need social connection in order to feel happy, we can use this to our advantage to help us stick to our habits.

When we tell someone that we are working to implement a positive habit, for example a new gratitude habit, our chances of sticking to it increase dramatically. By converting this intention from just a thought in our mind to something we've shared with another, we are far more likely to follow through. When you're selecting those habits that you want to try to embed, tell someone about them, whether it's a friend, a partner or your child. By communicating it to others you are sharing your vision and they'll support you by keeping you accountable and on track!

Let's take the example of you deciding that electronics before bed are negatively impacting your sleep. The habit that you want to implement is to stop looking at your phone before bed and read a book instead. This sounds easier than it is (I know from personal experience!) because of thoughts like 'but what if that person I am waiting to hear back from emails me?' or 'what if I could just check Instagram . . . ?', or whatever it might be. These thoughts then affect our feelings – in this case FOMO(!) – and then, in turn, our actions are that we take the phone with us to bed, just in case. However, if you agree with your partner that they'll be your accountability partner and that you'll both leave your phones charging downstairs when you go to bed and not look at them until the morning, you're far more likely to stick to it.

In the context of your child, if they have decided that they want to work towards riding their bike, for example, why not arrange for them to do it with a friend? The commitment to their friend will help them to get started and to keep going! If you're working towards any habit and you have an accountability partner, you are much more likely to stick to it and so much more likely to convert this into a habit.

Having an accountability partner doesn't mean that they have to do the activity with you – just telling someone that you're working towards this new habit has the same impact. It could be a friend that you ask to call you every Friday afternoon and remind you not to get that takeaway tonight! The point is that forming a social connection around the habit you're implementing will positively impact your ability to achieve it.

Getting an Action Plan in Place

In this final section I'm going to give you some time and space to think about the areas that you feel are most important to your family given what you've learnt. Remember at the very start of the book I said I'd be giving you an a la carte menu that you can choose from? Well, this is where you get to do the choosing!

I hope in reading the book to this point that you've had some 'Aha!' moments and have been able to recognise which areas resonated most strongly for you. Maybe you can see that your child really needs some help building their self-esteem. Or that they need support to manage their big emotions.

Learning to tune in and listen to those feelings is all part of fine-tuning that superpower you have of your parental intuition. You know your family best and you know what your child needs the most right now.

As you go through the next few pages, I am going to ask you to summarise your learnings and 'Aha!' moments and then commit to one thing that you're going to do differently in each area. Feel free to write, doodle or draw your reflections – whatever works best for you! If you want to add more things, that is great, but starting with one thing is really important in order to stop that overwhelm in its tracks. If you try to take on too much too soon, it will be harder for you to make any of it stick. Start small and build from there.

You may find it easier to flick back through the chapters at this point to remind yourself of what you wrote down in the key learnings section of each one. This will jog your memory and remind you of just how much you've learnt!

OK, let's start turning those 'Aha!' moments into action plans!

Meet Your Brain

My biggest learnings

....

....

....

....

....

....

....

....

How this can help my family

....

....

....

....

....

....

....

....

....

The one thing I am going to commit to trying is:

....

....

....

....

....

Here is how I will use situational support to do this:

....

....

....

....

....

Here is how I will use an accountability partner to help me:

....

....

....

....

....

Celebrate

My biggest learnings

....

....

....

....

....

....

....

....

How this can help my family

....

....

....

....

....

....

....

....

....

Putting It All Together

The one thing I am going to commit to trying is:

....
....
....
....
....

Here is how I will use situational support to do this:

....
....
....
....
....

Here is how I will use an accountability partner to help me:

....
....
....
....
....

Appreciate

My biggest learnings

....

....

....

....

....

....

....

....

How this can help my family

....

....

....

....

....

....

....

....

....

The one thing I am going to commit to trying is:

....

....

....

....

....

Here is how I will use situational support to do this:

....

....

....

....

....

Here is how I will use an accountability partner to help me:

....

....

....

....

....

Relate

My biggest learnings

....

....

....

....

....

....

....

....

How this can help my family

....

....

....

....

....

....

....

....

....

Putting It All Together

The one thing I am going to commit to trying is:

....

....

....

....

....

Here is how I will use situational support to do this:

....

....

....

....

....

Here is how I will use an accountability partner to help me:

....

....

....

....

....

Engage

My biggest learnings

....

....

....

....

....

....

....

....

How this can help my family

....

....

....

....

....

....

....

....

....

Putting It All Together

The one thing I am going to commit to trying is:

....

....

....

....

....

Here is how I will use situational support to do this:

....

....

....

....

....

Here is how I will use an accountability partner to help me:

....

....

....

....

....

CONCLUSION
Some Final Thoughts

You now have an action plan and you're ready to start implementing the parts of the myHappymind system that you feel are most relevant for you and your family right now. You've identified the areas that you need to focus on the most and now it's time to get started. Are you feeling excited? I hope so!

Before you jump in, though, can we just take a moment to reflect on the journey you've been on as you've read this book? You committed yourself to learning and growing, you've done the work and you're now ready to go and start taking action.

I want to take a moment to fully acknowledge you and your awesomeness! This work isn't easy. It can bring up all sorts of emotions and feelings, some of hope and excitement, some of fear and worry, but that is all totally normal. It just means you're in the learning zone, which is where you need to be to grow.

The fact that you're here and that you've reflected and considered and made some commitments means that you are so ready to start building your child's resilience, self-esteem and, ultimately, their happiness. Nothing brings me more joy than helping other parents fast-track through the process of learning how to build their child's confidence, but I understand that it can feel incredibly challenging at times.

I want to remind you of a few things before you go ahead and get started.

In *The Light in the Heart* Roy T. Bennett said, 'The one who falls and gets up is stronger than the one who never tried. Do not fear failure, but rather fear not trying.'

Trying new things can be hard, we don't always get them right the first time, but it is when we fail that we learn and grow. Please don't let any negative self-talk or fear stop you from having a go with these strategies. There is no race and no competition. All you need to focus on is doing a little bit better than yesterday – it really is that simple. If you try the gratitude habit and your child can't think of anything the first time you have the conversation, that's OK – they can try again next time. If you try to actively listen to your partner at the end of the day and you find yourself drifting off to check your phone, that's OK, you can try again next time. This isn't about chasing perfection, it is about making small but intentional attempts each and every day. This is your journey and what matters is that you try.

Some Final Thoughts

In her book, *The Gifts of Imperfection* Brené Brown said, 'When we deny our stories they define us. When we own our stories, we get to write a brave new ending.'

Here's the reality – we all tell ourselves stories about the way things are and the way they are supposed to be. Whether we're aware of them or not, we tell them. We also all have a story about how we were parented or how we've parented our children to this point. Whether these stories align with what you've learnt in the myHappymind system or not, it's time to write your own story about how you move forward from here. Whatever that story may be, it is crucial that you own it because you can write whatever story you want – you can move on from this point however you want to. Just make sure that the steps you take are conscious and that you're living the story you want to write, not the story that you may be telling yourself subconsciously.

Randy Pausch author of *The Last Lecture* said, 'Put on your own oxygen mask before assisting others.'

While if we were on a plane we know it would make sense to put on our own mask before we help our child with their own, I wonder how many of us actually would. The instinct to care for them first before we start to look after ourselves is so powerful that I'm just not sure how many of us as parents would be able to resist it.

Lucky for us we're not on a plane and we don't need to worry about oxygen masks! But we do have the time to take a moment here to stop and reflect on the extent to which you are looking after yourself. Because here's the truth – if we're not looking after our own mental health and happiness, it's really hard for us to teach our children to look after theirs.

If you feel that you aren't looking after yourself as much as you could then here's what I recommend. Start using the habits that you've learnt about in the myHappymind system on yourself first. Take some time to just start building your own resilience, your own self-esteem and your own relationships. Doing this will mean that you're putting your oxygen mask on first, which in turn will mean that you can better support your child. You will be so much more effective as a teacher if you're OK. So – this is me giving you full permission to put your oxygen mask on first. Nothing bad will happen to your little one if you invest this time in you.

If you're feeling good and ready to go then dive in! Just remember that you're in a learning zone and there will be bumps along the road. But something tells me that you've got this – I believe in you.

Lovely Notes

....
....
....
....
....
....
....
....
....
....
....
....
....
....

My Happy Mind

Lovely Notes

....

....

....

....

....

....

....

....

....

....

....

....

....

....

....

....

....

....

....

....

....

My Happy Mind

....
....
....
....
....
....
....
....
....
....
....
....
....
....
....
....
....
....
....
....
....

About myHappymind

myHappymind is an organisation dedicated to helping schools, nurseries, families and organisations teach resilience, self-esteem and mental well-being habits. We have a range of courses to support teachers, parents, children and individuals to develop these skills and provide a community for parents to connect, learn and grow.

If you'd like to learn more, check us out at myHappymind.org and follow me on Instagram and Facebook by searching for @myHappymind.

Digital resources

To access the digital resources in the book, all you need to do is go to: myHappymind.org/Bookgoodies and you can get your hands on them.

Acknowledgements

It is hard to know where to start in acknowledging all of the incredible people who have helped me on the journey to develop the myHappymind system and, ultimately, to write this book.

I have been fortunate to learn a tremendous amount from many of the psychologists and experts I mention throughout the book, and I am grateful for their wisdom, their research and their passion. I must also acknowledge all of my students, whether they are children, teachers or parents. Their inspiring stories of success and their commitment to their children's mental health is wonderful to watch and motivates me to keep sharing the myHappymind system.

I simply wouldn't have felt called to do this work if it were not for my family. My wonderful parents have always encouraged me to follow my dreams and passions – and continue to do so – and they've instilled in me a sense of resilience and self-belief that means I never fear a challenge! Their care, love and life of service to others has always been an inspiration and I'm grateful to have been raised by parents who taught me to work hard and to be kind. I feel lucky beyond words to be their daughter. To my brothers, whom I can probably credit some of my toughness to; growing up as the youngest with two older brothers will do that! Thank you for your care, love and support.

My own children, Oscar and Bella, were the inspiration behind myHappymind and continue to remind me why I do this work every single day. They both, in their own ways, carry a resilience and kindness that I am so proud to watch develop and grow. I can't even count the number of times they've told me they are proud of me or they've said 'don't worry' when I have to work. They've both had their fair share of challenges even at their young ages and I've been so proud of their kindness, resilience and love in dealing with them.

There have been many others who've supported me along the way, but special mention has to go to some of my 'mummy' friends who I admire and learn from all of the time. Susie, Franny, Lou, Bingum and so many more – you know who you are and thank you for your support, laughter, love and childcare when I've needed it!

And last but not least, to Tim, my loyal husband, who, unlike me, isn't a risk-taker but who always has my back,

Acknowledgements

always believes in me and always lets me pursue my passions even when they seem a little wild! Thank you for your unwavering support and patience as I have built myHappymind and for allowing me the time and space to write this book.

References

Preface

1 Kessler, R. C., Berglund, P., Demler, O., Jin, R., Merikangas, K. R. and Walters, E. E., 'Lifetime prevalence and age-of-onset distributions of DSM-IV disorders in the National Comorbidity Survey Replication.' *Archives of General Psychiatry* 62.6 (2005): 593–602.

2 Kessler, R. C., McLaughlin, K. A., Green, J. G., Gruber, M. J., Sampson, N. A., Zaslavsky, A. M., Aguilar-Gaxiola, S., Alhamzawi, A. O., Alonso, J., Angermeyer, M. and Benjet, C., 'Childhood adversities and adult psychopathology in the WHO World Mental Health Surveys.' *The British Journal of Psychiatry* 197.5 (2010): 378–85.

Chapter 2 Celebrate: Understanding Character

1 The VIA Institute on Character, 'The VIA Character Strengths Survey', https://viacharacter.org (accessed 8 Jul. 2020).

2 Seligman, M. E. and Csikszentmihalyi, M. (2000). 'Positive psychology: An introduction.' *American Psychologist* 55.1: 5–14.

3 Seligman, M. E., *Authentic Happiness: Using the new positive psychology to realize your potential for lasting fulfilment* (Simon & Schuster, 2004).

4 Waters, L., 'Why it's important to see and nurture the best in your child', The VIA Institute on Character, 13 May 2019, retrieved from https://www.viacharacter.org/topics/articles/why-its-important-to-see-and-nurture-the-best-in-your-child (accessed 8 Jul. 2020).

Chapter 3 Appreciate: Gratitude

1 McCullough, M. E. and Emmons, R. A., 'Counting blessings versus burdens: An experimental investigation of gratitude and subjective well-being in daily life.' *Journal of Personality and Social Psychology* 84.2 (2003): 377–89.

2 Seligman, M. E., Steen, T. A., Park, N. and Peterson, C., 'Positive psychology progress: Empirical validation of interventions.' *American Psychologist* 60.5 (2005): 410–21.

3 Van Boven, L. and Gilovich, T., 'To do or to have? That is the question.' *Journal of Personality and Social Psychology* 85.6 (2003): 1193–202.

4 Kumar, A., Killingsworth, M. A. and Gilovich, T., 'Waiting for merlot: Anticipatory consumption of experiential and material purchases.' *Psychological Science* 25.10 (2014): 1924–31.

5 Jose, P. E., Lim, B. T. and Bryant, F. B., 'Does savoring increase happiness? A daily diary study.' *The Journal of Positive Psychology* 7.3 (2012): 176–87.

Chapter 4 Relate: Building Positive Relationships

1 Myers, D. G., 'The funds, friends, and faith of happy people.' *American Psychologist* 55.1 (2000): 56.

2 Diener, E. and Seligman, M. E., 'Very happy people.' *Psychological Science* 13.1 (2002): 81–4.

References

3 Epley, N., *Mindwise: Why we misunderstand what others think, believe, feel, and want* (Vintage, 2015).

4 Boothby, E. J., Clark, M. S. and Bargh, J. A., 'Shared experiences are amplified.' *Psychological Science* 25.12 (2014): 2209–16.

Chapter 5 Engage: The Power of Goal-Setting and Dreaming

1 Klein, H. J., Whitener, E. M. and Ilgen, D. R., 'The role of goal specificity in the goal-setting process.' *Motivation and Emotion* 14.3 (1990): 179–93.

2 Stadler, G., Oettingen, G. and Gollwitzer, P. M., 'Intervention effects of information and self-regulation on eating fruits and vegetables over two years.' *Health Psychology* 29.3 (2010): 274–83.

Chapter 6 Putting It All Together

1 Ackerman, C. E., 'What is neuroplasticity? A psychologist explains', *Positive Psychology*, 28 Apr. 2020. retrieved from https://positivepsychology.com/neuroplasticity/ (accessed 8 Jul. 2020).

2 Painter, J. and Wansink, B., 'How visibility and convenience influence candy consumption.' *Appetite* 38.3 (2002): 237–8.

Index

Page references in *italics* indicate images.

Index

Index

Index

Index

Index

Index

About the Author

Laura Earnshaw worked as a Global HR Executive for 15 years helping leaders thrive under pressure and teams fulfil their potential. She's worked at Harvard Business School and with CEOs in the FTSE 100. After a friend close to her was sectioned under the mental health act, she quit her corporate job and set up myHappymind to help schools find a solution to the mental health problem. myHappymind is already being used by over 250,000 children, teachers and parents and is due to be taken up by the NHS and made available in 40 schools and 322 nurseries.